KU-020-565

Babe Bible

ESSENTIAL ADVICE ON EVERYTHING YOU NEED TO KNOW

Anita Naik

PIATKUS

*For Melanie McFadyean, who taught me
how to give advice and when to stand
back and take it.*

The opinions and advice expressed in this book are
intended as a guide only. Neither the publisher nor
the author is engaged in rendering professional
advice or services to the individual reader. If you
have a medical condition or are pregnant, the diet
and exercises described in this book should not be
followed without your first consulting your doctor.
The publisher and author accept no responsibility
for any injury or loss sustained as a result of the use
of this book.

Copyright © 2004 by Anita Naik
www.anitanaik.co.uk

First published in 2004 by
Piatkus Books Ltd
5 Windmill Street
London W1T 2JA

e-mail: info@piatkus.co.uk
The moral right of the author has been asserted

Reprinted 2005

A catalogue record for this book is available from
the British Library

ISBN 0 7499 2516 7

Text design by Briony Chappell
Edited by Jan Cutler
Illustrations by Robyn Neild

This book has been printed on paper manufactured
with respect for the environment using wood from
managed sustainable resources

Printed and bound in Great Britain by
CPI Bath

Visit the Piatkus website!

Piatkus publishes a wide range of best-selling fiction and
non-fiction, including books on health, mind, body & spirit,
sex, self-help, cookery, biography and the paranormal.

If you want to:
- read descriptions of our popular titles
- buy our books over the Internet
- take advantage of our special offers
- enter our monthly competition
- learn more about your favourite Piatkus authors

VISIT OUR WEBSITE AT: www.piatkus.co.uk

Anita Naik is a freelance writer who writes for *New Woman, Eve, Zest, Red, Cosmopolitan* and *Glamour*. Specialising in health, relationship and lifestyle issues, Anita was also the advice columnist on *Just 17* and *B* magazine, and is currently the advice columnist and health editor on *Closer* magazine.

Anita is also the author of:

The Lazy Girl's Guide to Beauty
The Lazy Girl's Guide to a Fabulous Body
The Lazy Girl's Guide to Good Health
The Lazy Girl's Guide to Good Sex
The Lazy Girl's Party Guide

Contents

Acknowledgements

With thanks to my wonderful agent Judy Chilcote, Helen Prangnell for all her research, and Jane N., Jenni B., Emma B., Alison I. and Leesa D. for endless advice and listening skills.

Introduction

'Common sense is not so common' — Voltaire

Advice – who needs it, especially from a stranger? Well, I'm with you there! After all, giving advice is just pure common sense, isn't it? Something anyone could do. Your best friend, your mother and even your boyfriend! Which means you could actually stop reading this book right now, stop feeling embarrassed and simply look at that sex book you really wanted to pick up in the first place. Advice – you see – it's everywhere, even when you're not even asking for it.

The truth is, thanks to modern life (and the fact that none of us has to be that worried with hunting-and-gathering issues) we're all busy looking for answers to the more irritating questions such as 'Why me?', 'How come?', and 'How the hell do I do that?'

Let's face it, life is at times hopelessly annoying, and if we're honest most of us are clinging on hoping that one disaster doesn't ricochet into a downward spiral of doom. Happy thoughts – no wonder there's no time to get fit, pay off your debts, find inner peace and still zap your bikini line every month. Most of us are lucky if we remember to get up and get dressed in the morning.

So, whether you find the answers to your problems in a coffee cup, in the arms of some gorgeous man or by living in a cave for a year, only you can say. All I can tell you is despite the fact that I make my living dishing out words of wisdom, like any good doctor I'm just another person who can't take my own medicine. Not only do I spend my days doing the utterly ridiculous, but also I can't give up coffee for my health, date normal men for my sanity, and convince myself of the point of doing yoga. Worse still, I don't own a sensible pair of shoes, have no idea how to change a tyre and won't eat fruit. And though my home looks calm and cool on the outside, open a cupboard and everything, including my knickers, will probably fall out. It's a messy, untidy world and there's no getting around that.

However, I do know from experience

that a bit of good advice can, and will, make all the difference. Not only in how you feel but also in what you can achieve and feel happy about, and by good advice I don't mean any old advice thrown your way.

'Learn to be discerning' is my best advice tip, and never ever follow gems such as 'Yes, it is a good idea to dance in heels on a bar stool/stand by a glass table when you're drunk.'

As for asking for advice, well there's nothing to be embarrassed about because the fact is whether you write to advice columns, bore strangers in bars, or obsess about your life with friends, asking for directions is normal. It's about gaining better information on how to make life easier. It's also, of course, about the semi-serious issues like finding out why people run screaming from a room when you come near them (BO, personality disorder or their problem?), and why when you earn a healthy wage you're still poorer than a church mouse (clue: you own more shoes than the population of Wales).

More importantly, advice is about reassurance. We all want and need to know we're good people at heart, especially when we snap at our loved ones, date guys who can't remember our names, and/or fall asleep every time a friend calls with yet another 'Why-am-I-single?/It's-because-I'm-fat/I'm-going-to-die-alone-aren't-I?' tale of woe. And this is where *Babe Bible* can help you, because all problems are relative, which means the answer to life's complexities are much simpler than you think.

At the core of every problem is someone who simply wants a way out, needs to feel better and hopes they can change their future and not repeat the past. As I said earlier, advice is simply the common sense you can't see when you're too busy falling apart. So after a lifetime of dishing it out (15 years, zillions of letters and ample personal mistakes, if you must know), I've thrown together the best life-saving gems to help you improve, fix, repair and gloss over the catastrophic events. Better still, it's all rolled into a self-help, bossy-best-friend, oracle-of-information handbook better known as: OK STOP WHINING AND CHANGE THINGS NOW. Take my advice: read this book – you won't regret it.

life

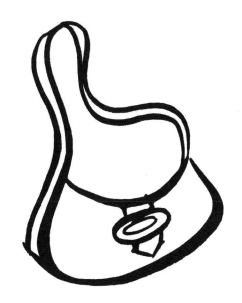

How to find your willpower

 Whatever your weakness – your loser ex, chocolate-covered doughnuts, pints of lager – the chances are when it comes to enforcing steely resolve to give up and stay away you just can't do it. For most of us, fighting temptation with willpower feels as impossible as going one round with Mike Tyson. The problem is that self-restraint is a double negative. Tell yourself you can't have something and all that happens is you want it even more. Here's what to do if you're feeling weak-willed.

Change your state

You know the score: it's 8.00 p.m., you've had dinner, you're not hungry, but the fridge is beckoning. All you can think of is the plate of leftovers, a packet of biscuits, and even a slice of cake. Your impulse is to eat, eat, eat, and you can't find the strength to stick to your diet – what's a girl to do? Apart from putting temptation out of reach (and in the bin outside), experts suggest changing your state, also known as: getting the hell away from your object of desire. Get up, go out, and run round to see a friend. Distracting yourself like this boosts willpower because it takes the focus off your urge, meaning you stop wanting it so much.

Visualise the repercussions

Desperate to call the ex who broke your heart and see him just one more time? You're lonely, it's late, he's willing – so why not? The only way out of this is to visualise what will happen post-meeting and then call your most stern friend and tell her your intentions. Mostly when we lose willpower we fool ourselves that we can handle the repercussions by glossing over the specifics. To boost willpower, you have to focus on the details.

Give yourself a pep talk

Willpower often flags when you keep reminding yourself of all the times you've failed in the past. What's important now is not how you failed in the past but how you'll succeed in the present. To get this thought to stick, learn from your mistakes. It wasn't just the concept of lack of willpower that made you fail before, but specifics. Do stress and upset play a part in your flagging willpower, or PMS or even lack of family support? Pinpoint your weak links and times, and work out ways you can override them.

Give yourself a break

Willpower disintegrates when you put yourself under what's known as an 'all-or-nothing' mentality. Instead, come up with a realistic plan that works long term for you. This should always include space to be 'naughty', whether that means a treat once a day, a pair of expensive running shoes to get you to the gym, or a mass flirting session to get your ex off your mind.

Babe pointers

+ **Put temptation out of reach** A simple but effective tool for boosting willpower. If you are trying to avoid drinking and smoking, don't go to the places where you used to smoke and drink for at least four weeks – the time it takes to break a habit.
+ **Have two objectives** First find yourself a long-term goal – one that's your ultimate objective – and then a short-term goal. Small achievements are as important as big ones because they keep you going and are a good way to measure ongoing success.
+ **Tell yourself you can do it** Don't surround yourself with people who laugh when you tell them what you're up to. You may have lost your willpower millions of times before, but who's to say you can't do it this time. Lots of people try 100 times until they reach their goal.
+ **Relax** Finally, don't let self-restraint take over your life – it's addictive when you get the hang of it, but unhealthy if you make it your whole purpose in life.

3

How to be on time

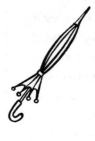

Always in a mad rush from A to B, constantly ten minutes (or more) late, feeling there are just not enough minutes in the day to do what needs to be done? Well, if it's any consolation, it's worth knowing that the world is divided into people who are always late and people who aren't. Natural disasters, emotional breakdowns and large traffic delays apart, being late is less about being too busy to get to places on time, and more about poor time management. So here's how never to be late again.

Look at where your time goes

If you're losing minutes and finding that time just slips through your fingers, it pays to account for your time in the same way you account for your money. Look at how and why your minutes slip away. Do you talk too long on the phone, get easily distracted by post, papers and people walking by? Are you disorganised and a last-minute doer who never accounts for realistic timings in your planning?

Be realistic about your time

Eager to keep everyone happy, have a great work life and still do the things you want? That's great except there are only 24 hours in the day and this means you need to be realistic about how long things take to do, and why. Trying to do everything is the key to chronic lateness, simply because struggling to squeeze everything in pushes time to its absolute limits and therefore leaves no safety zone for factors you have no control over, such as traffic and transport.

Factor in 15 minutes extra

It's no good hoping for a best-case scenario every time, because life has a way of throwing a spanner in the works. Always give yourself ten to 15 minutes extra with every task and appointment you've scheduled in. 'Expect the best and prepare for the worst' is probably the best motto for getting to places on time.

Prioritise

With this in mind, it's sensible therefore to prioritise what's essential and important and what isn't on a day-to-day basis. The aim is to plan your time so that the important tasks are achieved with time to spare, and the rest is stored for another day. To help yourself do this, make lists; this will not only help you keep track of things, but also give you a clear indication of your obligations.

Avoid the 'one-last-thing' scenario

This is the thing you see when you're just about to the leave the house. It could be something as mundane as putting the rubbish out, calling your mother or filing something, but the problem is you think it will take a minute although it will really take ten minutes or more (thereby blowing your emergency time zone). Forget about it and just leave already!

If desperate, set an alarm

As jangling as this is on your nerves, alarms work because they shake you out of your current state and make you aware that you now have to move on to something else.

Babe pointers

+ **Time is precious for everyone** Don't think an apology for being late will always suffice.
+ **Delegate at work** Chronic lateness at work (whether it's for meetings or for deadlines) is usually a symptom that you haven't delegated properly.
+ **Pay attention to details** It sounds simple, but most people who can't deal with time rarely have a watch, look at a clock or read the small print. Don't assume you know things like the directions to a place or the address and/or even the meeting time – check these things out in advance so you're not caught out at the last minute.
+ **It's not a genetic problem** Don't fool yourself about your timekeeping and say you can't help it. If you can get to a first date on time, manage to get to a shoe shop before it closes – you can get to places on time.

How to get rich

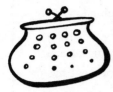

Apart from marrying a millionaire, inventing a way to get thin without dieting, or winning the lottery, getting rich is all about financial strategy. If your current strategy involves throwing your bank statements unopened into the bin, shopping for clothes rather than eating, and knowing the guaranteed way to buy shoes without having your credit card rejected, you need a new strategy. The good news is: just because you have zero savings, and no chance of a distant relative leaving you a hidden fortune, it doesn't mean you can't one day be rich. However, it takes planning, it takes saving and it takes a financial game plan. Here's how.

Start saving now

Studies show that most of us can save a good percentage of our monthly wage if we break it down in our minds. Think of a lump sum you want to save and then divide it by 30 to see how much this works out to be on a day-by-day basis. Small savings equal big long-term dividends.

Shop sensibly

Don't be a sucker for the adverts selling you a lifestyle through packaging. Shop wisely by picking the right store to shop in (not all supermarkets are created equal). More importantly, pay attention to in-house deals, shop on the Internet for cheaper bargains, buy during the sales, and work on the basis that if you have two white T-shirts you don't need one more.

Direct debit your savings

Saving can actually be as addictive as buying once you watch the numbers crunch upwards. If you don't trust yourself to save each month, take the decision out of your hands by direct debiting your savings the moment you get paid.

Think long-term and short-term portfolios

Ask any financial expert (or rich person) and they'll tell you they have a variety of savings based on short-term, mid-term and long-term goals. Long term should be a pension, for retirement, whereas mid term is for a house – or getting fired! Short term should be for holidays or savings to buy a car, TV, or fancy outfit.

Take measured risks

As tempting as it is to dabble in the stock market, or invest in a pyramid-selling scheme and give your money to someone who says they can triple it in two weeks, there's a phrase worth considering: if it sounds too good to be true – it is! No one gets rich quick unless they can afford to lose money – and if you're someone who isn't currently rich you can't afford to take risks with your hard-earned wages.

Buy a property

Still the best long-term investment you can make as long as you don't overstretch yourself, borrow against it or hope to double your money in a year. On average, aim to stay in your house for three to five years and get yourself a mortgage you can afford.

Babe pointers

+ **Everything counts** Pick a credit card with no interest to pay back, and a current account that gives you interest, alongside your savings. The small stuff does count in the long run. Likewise, watching what you buy in the supermarket may only save you a small amount a week but this can add up to a large saving over a year!
+ **Make spending hard** Credit-card spending fools us all into thinking we're not really spending cash. Help yourself by cutting up your cards or not taking them out with you so you can avoid spontaneous (read: too expensive for me) buys.
+ **Lose the treat mentality** This is the thinking that actually gives you permission to spend more than you make. You don't need a treat for lowering your debt, eating at home for a whole week and/or saving money. The treat is one day you'll be rich!
+ **Budget** Otherwise known as: stop dreaming and get real, and make a concrete plan that's going to get you from zero to a million in 20 years.

How to be less judgemental

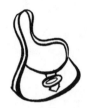

Life – it's full of things just waiting to be criticised, isn't it? The state of the country, the way people drive/live/eat/speak, who's dating whom and even why the heck that person thought they looked good in that outfit when they so obviously didn't! In fact being judgemental has become a bit of a national pastime – just check out any newspaper or TV show to see.

The problem is that criticism of others, especially of the vicious and non-constructive variety, reflects our own level of insecurity. Attack someone for basically ruining their relationship/eating badly and having a bottom the size of China and all you're doing is giving yourself permission to feel smug about your own choices, no matter how unhappy they make you or how wrong you secretly feel they are. Likewise, slating others for their

mistakes, weaknesses and flaws is simply another way not to feel so bad when we mess up (because let's face it, there's always someone messing up more spectacularly than us).

Why we are critical

Research shows that the wobblier we are about our own lives, and decisions, the more we are likely to criticise others. Which means if you're judgemental to the hilt, the chances are you're also super hard on your own decisions and choices. The cure, therefore, couldn't be simpler – give others (and yourself) a break. So what if someone is taking a different road to you and making a choice that jars your senses? What real difference does it make to your life?

No one likes bitchiness

Self-reflection aside, one good reason not to spend your time judging others is simply that no one wants to be around a person who is down on everyone else all the time. Not only is it dull but also it screams of spite, anger and viciousness – not qualities that most people look for in a friend and/or lover. Of course, while we do live in a world where success is measured by comparison, such as how fast, clever and basically more attractive we are than others, there will always be people who fall both above and below you. Meaning it's all a huge waste of time. Instead of getting irritated by other people's choices, let it go and just get on with your own life.

Babe pointers

+ **Break the habit** Being critical is a habit, and the more you do it the more it becomes second nature. Take your mum's advice: if you've got nothing nice to say, don't say anything. To break the bitch cycle, check yourself. Think before you speak, and consciously make yourself say something positive, every time you feel a criticism coming on.
+ **Don't use criticisms to bond** Being judgemental is contagious and it's often tempting to use a nasty comment to get someone to like you.

It works but it's a short term remedy if your aim is to make real friends.
+ **Don't be afraid to express a good opinion** Standing up to people's harsh judgements of others and offering a different point of view can be hard, but it's a good way to boost your self-confidence and gain a more positive reputation from others.
+ **What are you excusing?** Can't stem the critical flow? Then you need to look at what you are excusing in yourself. Judgemental about a person's eating habits? Then ask yourself what it is about your own habits that their behaviour is triggering for you?
+ **Get rid of your pedestal mentality** Place someone above you and it's only a matter of time before they plummet to earth. On the whole, when we want someone to do something for us, such as make us feel happy, safe, or even secure, and it doesn't happen, most of us will retaliate in a critical way. To avoid being judgemental, simply avoid imposing your expectations and world-view on others.

How to stop procrastinating

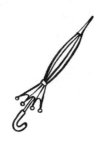

If you're someone who constantly postpones the inevitable, makes excuses about why your amazingly brilliant idea can't or won't work, or talks furiously about what you are going to do but lets your plans fade out when it's time to put them into action – you're a procrastinator! Unsure if this is you, or procrastinating about your status? Well here's a clue. If your friends' eyes glaze over when you come up with yet another grand scheme, and/or laugh loudly in the face of another of your business/relationship/holiday ideas, then the chances are you've procrastinated one time too many.

Face your home truths

The simple truth is: procrastinating is all about the fear of failure; it's not about pondering your options and letting them take their time to bloom. Procrastinating is the excuse factory in your head, which convinces you it's OK to dither and wait, rather than take action and do something.

Home truth number one Pure luck, osmosis and winning the lottery are not realistic ways to put your plans into action.

Home truth number two People don't take procrastinators seriously on a long-term basis, which means it does your professional and social profile no good.

Home truth number three Procrastinating is not the same as planning! Planning is an active word – it stirs you into action, helps you make plans and takes you on the first step towards your goal.

Home truth number four Be honest about why you're procrastinating. Here's how:

Three simple steps to success

1 **Ask yourself why.** No one repeats a pattern that doesn't bring him or her some kind of reward. For instance, are you hooked on the thrill of what could be – rather than discovering what the reality could be? Unsurprising because the thrill

of 'What if ... ?' is always more enticing than the hard work of getting from A to B.

2 **Change your thinking.** It's easier than you think, if you change your focus. Instead of imagining all the potential mistakes you could make, think right now about all the possible gains you will make (such as you won't always be living in the future and can start to live in the present).

3 **Take action.** Otherwise known as: do something besides talk. To actually get started, select a time zone of just ten minutes and sit down and make a plan. If your aim is to lose weight, begin by breaking the idea down into six practical goals, two of which you should be able to do right now. Next, work out what you're going to do tomorrow, the next day, and so on, as the key here is to keep the momentum going, and – bingo! you're no longer procrastinating.

Babe pointers

✦ **Don't spend your life being a big talker** Big talkers rarely achieve their goals, simply because all their energy is spent discussing rather than doing. Don't let excuses hold you back. If you don't have the money, think about how you could raise a loan.

✦ **Don't focus on your past failures** Mistakes aren't failures if you learn where you went wrong. The more full attempts you make to do something, the higher your chances of success.

✦ **Learn to take small steps** Don't be a speed freak – if an idea's worth pursuing it will take time to get there. To help yourself, share your goals with two people you respect (studies show we're more motivated when we feel obliged to do something).

✦ **Set yourself a time limit** If you haven't got the time, get up one hour earlier each day. If you are still dithering, let your idea go and find a new one. Remember: the most successful people have the same 24 hours as you do.

How to change

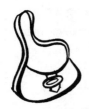

Can a leopard really change its spots? 'No,' says most of the population, suspicious about the whole idea of a person's ability to change. Yet, the fact remains that most of us would like to kick back against our past and become a new person, and why shouldn't we? Well, despite the adage that no one changes, people change all the time; not only physically but also mentally, and certainly in the way they choose to behave. You may be thinking: why even bother to change? Well, one good reason is that change can have an amazing effect on your whole life. If you're unhappy, fed up, miserable or just sick of yourself, a change is as good as a rest. It beats hours spent navel-gazing and time spent whingeing to your friends. Here's how to do it.

Work out what's got to change and why

Often when we're unhappy we think our whole lives are a waste of time and energy. We imagine that if only we were far off on a desert island away from the crowds things would be better, because we could be who we truly are. The reality is you can't take a holiday from yourself. When you talk about change, you're essentially talking about making different choices that will make your life happier and fuller. These are choices about the way you're living, whom you spend time with, your health, your job and even your mindset.

Don't let trauma drive you

Studies show we always change in the midst or the aftermath of a trauma: a broken heart, a period of depression, bereavement or even an illness. While this can be a good thing, it's important that you don't let this be your only driving force towards change. Many a deep end has been jumped into with regret. Slow down before you do anything that appears rash to others, and ask a trusted friend for their advice.

Remember: good things can change you too. Success and love can transform your life, as can the right job, the right city or even the right book. So ask yourself: if you could have anything, what's the one thing that would transform you right now? And go for it.

You can change right now

Change isn't necessarily a process that takes time; sometimes it can be instantaneous. However, it is an ongoing process and one where the goal posts should regularly move. To start, write a list of things you want to change in order of preference, starting with what you need to change first; put the three things you would have to do today at the top, to set this in motion. Next reinforce the change by ensuring you do something towards it every day. For example, if you want to move from fat to fit, do some form of exercise each day to reinforce the idea that you're changing and are a different person from the day before.

Babe pointers

+ **Nothing stays the same** You may want to stay in the same place and would prefer for nothing to change, but change occurs every day, little by little, so you have to embrace it or you simply get left behind.
+ **Don't be afraid of change** Change isn't difficult but the period of transformation is. Anything new feels uncomfortable for a while, and it takes time to get used to new behaviours, a new look, or even new insights into your life. Give yourself a month to get used to something before you consider tinkering with it.
+ **Ask for help** No woman is an island! Ask for help, advice and support as you change. You'll be surprised at how many people will want to help.
+ **Change the right things** Sometimes a superficial change is all you'll need to feel recharged; other times change has to come from within. What is worth considering is that any change, no matter how small, triggers a domino effect.

How to de-clutter

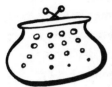Is your life a mess? We're not talking metaphors here, but a literal mess, in the sense: are you a bit of a domestic slut? Disorderly conduct is now as normal as domestic bliss was in the 1950s, and most houses are now so cluttered with possessions – gadgets and clothes – that most people would rather move house than attempt to de-clutter. Fancy decors and feng-shui theories apart, it makes sense to clear up your rubbish simply to give yourself some physical space in your home. Here's how to make your home an oasis of calm.

Be honest

Your house is a mess because you're untidy. You may be clean, you may know what a vacuum cleaner is, but if your place looks like it's been robbed it's simply because you haven't picked up after yourself. Clutter is not just a mass of things, but a sign that you've let your possessions overwhelm you. This means it's the direct result of being slack, disorganised and generally lazy about the way you live.

Look at what you're dealing with

Start by sorting out one room at a time, and stick to that room so you're not tempted to spread the clutter further. Label four bin bags with the words: Dump, Keep, Give away, and Store.

Don't be sentimental

Be ruthless – you don't have to keep birthday cards because friends and family sent you them. Also throw or give away books you don't read any more, holiday pictures you've only looked at once (if they're not in an album you won't look at them anyway), empty plastic and carrier bags, gifts you dislike and magazines and papers that are more than a month old. If in doubt ask yourself why you're keeping them – and if you haven't got two good reasons, throw them out. With precious objects that do have sentimental value, ask yourself why you haven't got them on show.

Enlist the help of a friend to sort out clothes

Most of us have way too many clothes, the result of fickle buys, overspending and generally not de-junking. To successfully de-clutter a wardrobe you need the help of a good friend. Take everything out and throw away anything you haven't worn in the last two years. Anything too small, too big, too out of fashion, too ugly or totally unworn should be on the 'Out' pile. Hoping to regain your figure from years ago? Give it up. Experts say it's hard to move on and accept yourself when you're still trying to be someone from your past.

Ditch the bags

You've cleaned up – now give yourself a deadline for getting rid of those bags of clutter. Countless times people fall down on the final hurdle of de-cluttering simply because they don't get round to taking bags to charity shops and ditching the rubbish. Then, to keep on top of your clutter every day, be realistic. Help yourself by having only one small clutter area, for example a table top where clutter can be deposited and left. Be strict, keep it to this area, and regularly go through it.

Babe pointers

+ **Be organised** Avoid just throwing things into a box. Be systematic about your clearing-and-storing technique, and mark boxes so you know where things are.
+ **Keep the things you like on hand** Keep frequently-used items in accessible areas to avoid having to unpack things again.
+ **Tidy and clear at the same time** Remember: de-cluttering is a two-directional process – one is to put things back in their proper place, and two is to throw away all the things you no longer need.
+ **Always keep your objective in mind** A peaceful and calm living environment is your aim – something that you won't have if you're wedged on the sofa between clean laundry, an overflowing cat-litter tray and a pile of old newspapers.

How to stop moaning

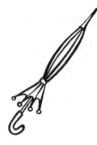

Moaning is not only tempting to do but weirdly enjoyable. Think about it: if we're not moaning about the weather, our financial status or our jobs, we're moaning about celebrities and their lives. The TV is at it, the newspapers, and even strangers we hardly know are more likely to strike up a conversation based on moans and complaints rather than on something good. Signs you are the moan queen of the year include: friends who suggest you might like to look on the bright side for a change; people asking if you ever say anything positive; and family members giving you helpful hints on how to be a glass-half-full kind of girl. The trouble with moaning is it's addictive, amusing (for a while) and easy to do because it takes virtually no effort. Unfortunately, the downside of this is it's downright depressing, and after a while it can turn you into a social leper. Here's what to do to save yourself from the moan zone.

Just stop moaning!

Yes, it's that easy! Just stop doing it by noticing how easily you slip into the habit of complaining. Tell yourself that today you aren't going to trash anyone, complain about public transport or generally get annoyed by things out of your control. If you can't manage a whole day, give yourself a time zone, or see if you can get through at least one conversation without moaning.

Do something about it

Of course, there are also legitimate things to moan about. The problem is, though, moaning is a passive action, as you tend to moan rather than do something to change the situation you're moaning about. So write that letter, call customer services, or confront someone about their unreasonable or unhelpful behaviour.

Break the habit

Be aware of how much you moan and then think how boring it must be for people around you to hear the same thing again and again. If you need to get it out, write it down. Then before you utter a moan, take ten seconds and a deep breath. The delay in getting the words out of your mouth should stop the action of actually moaning and give you the brain space to think of something more positive to say.

Put a positive spin on things

For every moan that comes to mind make a conscious effort to put a positive spin on it! Finding an alternative in your mind is the way to turn from a complainer into someone more positive. Remind yourself of the rewards of this type of communication. In the workplace it will give you better standing with the management, as it will allow them to see you as a motivator. Socially, your friends will not only feel more uplifted around you but also be more inclined to come to you for support (moaning in sympathy is not positive support).

Babe pointers

+ **Allow yourself three moans a day** Because, let's face it, it's impossible to go cold turkey, and sometimes it's a case of better out than in. However, choose wisely and make sure your complaints give you the release you're looking for.
+ **Don't become Pollyanna** There's nothing worse than a born-again positivity freak; while it's good to break the moan habit, don't swap one habit for another.
+ **Consider how it makes you feel** If you just can't stop the stream of moans, then consider how moaning makes you feel about yourself and your life. Studies have shown that constant moaning lowers mood and increases fatigue levels.
+ **Instigate forgiveness** As in, don't hold on to your gripes. Sometimes friends let us down, bosses are useless and promises are broken – that's life. Instead of moaning about it, forgive and move on – it's far simpler than grumbling your life away.

How to lose your couch-potato status

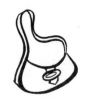 OK, let's be honest here – if you have a reputation as a couch potato it's likely this exists for a number of reasons: (1) because you are; (2) because you tend to let everyone know you are; and (3) because you quite enjoy the notoriety of it all. But we're not just talking about someone whose idea of exercise is walking from the sofa to the fridge and back, or a person who prefers to watch TV to going out, we're talking … laziness. Yes, sadly if you're known as the best couch potato in town, what your friends and family are basically saying is that they consider you to be incredibly lazy. To change your status, consider the following.

Change your habits

'Habits' as in 'horrible habits': smoking, drinking too much and surviving on pizza are the habits of a couch potato. Interject some healthy parts into your unhealthy bits, and you will not only feel better but also look better and maybe even feel like hauling yourself vertical every now and then.

Change your diet

Lack of energy and fatigue are the number-one reasons why people head for the comfort of their couch the second they get home and find they have no energy to do more active things. The answer is to eat more of the food your mother always told you to eat – fruit, vegetables, wholemeal bread, meat and fish, and less junk, ready-made and sugar-based meals.

Exercise

If you're someone who once hated PE lessons, the chances are the only times you think about trainers are as a fashion item, and exercise is something only the insane do. However, the fastest way to lose your couch-potato tag is to get fit, or at least make an attempt to get fit.

More good news is that exercise is cumulative. Do it in ten-minute spurts every hour you're at home (morning and evening) and by the end of the day you should have 60 minutes under your belt.

Change your behaviour

Lazy people have one essential habit that active people don't have – and that's the ability to let other people actively do things for them. Meaning there's no quicker and more pleasing a way to get rid of your couch-potato tag than to take the initiative and do something.

Babe pointers

+ **Work out what's keeping you inert** Is it lack of ideas, lack of confidence and/or lack of energy? If so, tackle one area at a time. No idea where to start? Buy a health magazine, join a gym, activate something with your friends. This will then increase your confidence. For lack of energy, look at your diet, your sleep patterns and whether or not it's laziness, rather than lack of energy.

+ **Motivate yourself** Of course, if you don't know why you're changing, you won't try to change, so find yourself a motivating factor. This could be to drop a dress size, shake up your life, feel better about your life, or simply to learn something new. Can't do it on your own? Well, enlist the help of either a super-active friend or a super-lazy one to do it with you.

+ **Give yourself a new label** Labels stick, but thankfully they are just as easy to peel off and rewrite. So instead of telling yourself you're lazy, change the record and give yourself a new tag. At the same time don't let people keep putting you in the same hole. So what if they don't believe you can change? What matters is what you think.

+ **Have some lazy times** There is a lot to be said for being lazy sometimes, so don't give it up entirely. It's good for the soul to know how and when to relax, and let's face it there's nothing better than spending the odd evening on the sofa.

How to get the life you want

Life – don't you just love it? So many opportunities to be happy, be successful, be loved up? If this isn't a reflection of your current state, don't despair. If you feel stuck on the course of your life, here's how to get the life you want.

Brainstorm

Make a list of what makes you happy. Think of all the things you have done, achieved and experienced, and even go back to your childhood and add the elements you once enjoyed. The point of this is to remind yourself of the areas you do get satisfaction out of – something that's easy to forget when you feel blue – or to help you work out which direction to take your life into.

Have a strategy

The next step is to prioritise a strategy list so that you have a clear indication of the elements that are most important to you. These could be: (1) love; (2) making money; (3) career; (4) having fun; (5) travelling; and so on – whatever variation feels the most right for you. Next, break down each of your goals into realistic steps that you can put into action right this second. For example, if it's a new career you're after, call up your local college, right now, for a prospectus; if it's love you're after, make arrangements to go out for the weekend and search for it.

Find a mentor

This is someone who is already where you want to be (or at least in the zone) and finding her or him is an essential part of attaining your life goals. Apart from showing you it can be done, you can learn a lot from someone already living the life you want.

Take yourself out of your comfort zone

Otherwise known as: challenge yourself. Life gets boring when you sit around being too comfortable – whether this is being in a job that pays well but no longer inspires you, or in a relationship that's easy but no longer holds any passion for you. Bear in mind that in order to live the life you want, you need uncertainty as well as certainty; too much of one or too little of the other and life is either too boring or too stressful.

Take risks

Just do it. Sometimes all the talking and planning in the world won't get you anywhere if you don't add action to the mix. Don't be too worried about making the right or wrong decision; just make a decision, because although that's the hardest step it's also the most important one.

Babe pointers

+ **Learn from your mistakes** In a study of super-millionaires, researchers found that the richest of the rich got there by taking responsibility for their mistakes instead of blaming others or circumstances beyond their control. The upshot of this is they: (1) felt in control of their lives and destiny; and (2) discovered where they had been going wrong.

+ **Take responsibility for your life** If you're not happy where you are, stop blaming others and start doing something about it. This might sound a bit New Agey, but life is what YOU make it. Don't let others or circumstances dictate where you are in life – be proactive and seek out change.

+ **Don't blame your parents** Otherwise known as: let go of the past. Life isn't easy and simple for everyone and, yes, some of us have more challenges and hurdles than others, and you're right – it's not fair. However, this isn't an excuse to stop trying – the past doesn't have to equal the future unless you let it.

+ **Change the record** You may have been a loser/failure/no-hoper yesterday, but this isn't you today, unless you keep sitting there and doing nothing!

you

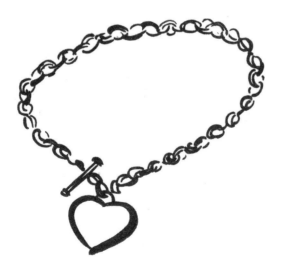

How to be happy

Are you one of those glass-half-full kind of girls – cheerfully optimistic in the face of any adversity? Graceful when life slaps you in the face? Overflowing with positivity and cheer, even to people who get on your nerves? Well, good for you if you are, because studies show that a cheerful disposition will get you through most of life's trials and tribulations. The key to happiness is, says a study from Harvard University: humour, caring for others, self-control, channelling your passions and planning ahead. Here's how to make happiness work for you.

Change your attitude

Happiness is a matter of perception; after all, two people can view the very same situation and end up with different emotional responses. While much of this is learnt behaviour from our parents (happy people tend to have been taught how to be happy rather than to have been born that way), it's never too late to change your attitude. What it takes is a conscious effort to look on the bright side and see the good in a situation and not the bad.

Forget about the lottery

Many people are convinced that if only they could win the lottery, find Mr Right, wake up thin, be famous or score all of the above then they would be happy. If you think like this it's worth noting that millionaires don't tend to smile any more than people living on the minimum wage. Happiness is an internal mindset and, although external factors affect our state of mind, lasting happiness comes from the way you tackle life, not from what life gives you.

Up your happiness score

We all set our own happiness score. Some people feel better when the sky is blue and the sun is shining, others when they're on holiday, and others still when a compliment has been thrown their way. If you rarely feel happy, then you need to up your score. Are you waiting for large events to transform your life? If so, work on feeling happy with the small ones.

Don't choose the dark side

Being cynical and dark as opposed to happy and optimistic doesn't make you a deeper or more intellectual person. What is more, nothing was ever made better by being miserable about it.

Learning to be grateful with what you have is a major key to living happily. It's OK to want more, strive for something better and hope that things improve, but at the same time don't devalue what you have. 'Be grateful' might sound like a parental admonishment but it's about seeing that while your life may not be perfect, it's your life so make it a happy one.

Babe pointers

+ **Don't compare your life with others'** The fastest way to feel unhappy is to look over your shoulder constantly and catalogue all the things that you haven't got but that your friends have. It's not about keeping up with anyone, but about choosing a life that's full of things that make you happy and content.

+ **Practise self-awareness not self-absorption** It's OK to look at how you respond to the world and analyse how and why you do things. However, being self-absorbed is a whole other board game. Don't immerse yourself in self-help books to the point that you can't do anything without overanalysing your actions. Sometimes it pays to just do it.

+ **Do something meaningful** Not necessarily VSO in a developing country, but actions and interests that hold meaning for you. Think about mentoring a child, doing a voluntary service for someone in your area, or offering your skills to a local school.

+ **Feel connected** A sense of belonging brings happiness because it makes you believe you have a place in the world. Make as many connections as you can with people you meet, whether it's at work, through friends, or even when you're in the gym.

How to be single

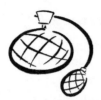

OK, you're probably thinking you don't need advice on this – after all, it wasn't your choice/idea/dream to be single. However, what this section is really about is how to be happily single (rather than happy that you're single). Of course, I'm not denying that on certain days there is a palpable feeling of emptiness and gloom about being single. Days when you're sure Mr Right is never going to appear and that somehow it's entirely your fault because you ate two chocolate bars and a packet of crisps for lunch. Being happily single isn't about pretending you don't have these feelings, it's about learning how to be happy on your own – something that everyone needs to learn, regardless of whether they are in love with someone or not. Remember: if you can't be happy on your own then you'll always be dependent on someone else for your happiness, and that's not a good recipe for a healthy relationship. Here's how to get the single thing right.

What's wrong with me?

You're single so something must be wrong with you, right? Well, wrong actually – not having a boyfriend doesn't mean that you're ugly, fat, unattractive and somehow fatally flawed. Go down this path and I guarantee that not only will you stay single (after all, how will anyone like you when you don't even like yourself?) but you'll also be miserable most of the time. Of course, it's never easy when someone asks, 'So, why are you single?' But the answer is not a passive 'No one's asked me out yet,' it's 'I haven't found someone I want to be with.'

All the best men are taken

Otherwise known as: all men are unfaithful/liars and/or incapable of commitment. While it is tempting and amusing at times to classify men in this way, if you sit about and condemn them all, you'll never notice when a good one comes along and stares you in the face. Plus, our brain believes what we tell it. Act down on men and you'll start thinking, 'What's the point of even trying to meet someone?'

Find the life you want

Which leads me nicely on to the fact that it's the women who lead happy and full lives who are more likely to meet the man of their dreams than the women who spend all their time looking. Learn to cultivate a life that you want by not only finding other interests besides dating but also surrounding yourself with people who do more than talk and complain about being single.

Learn to love other things besides men

Not only is this a good way to find a sense of purpose in your life (and it's worth noting that saying marriage is your only purpose is particularly pitiful) but also it will help you to see that, single or attached, you can live a wonderful and full life.

Babe pointers

✦ **You're lucky to be a single woman** According to studies, single women are not only healthier, richer and happier than single men but they also fare better than married women and end up living longer, so what are you complaining about?

✦ **Don't be afraid to say you're looking** Just because you're happy being a single girl doesn't mean you can't look or tell people you're looking for love. Ask friends to set you up, go on blind dates, and try Internet dating, the personals and speed dating. It doesn't mean you're desperate, it means you're open to anything.

✦ **Don't feel sorry for yourself** You're single, not sad – keep repeating this mantra to yourself especially in those dark-teatime-of-the-soul moments when you feel that you're going to be single and alone for ever.

✦ **Stop thinking life would be perfect if you had a boyfriend** It's nice when you're in love but it certainly isn't a stress-free zone.

How to boost your self-esteem

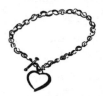

Feel that you're rubbish at everything, unattractive, too fat or too thin (even though everyone says you're not), and not as clever/witty and charming as everyone else you know? If so, you have what's known as low self-esteem. It sounds like a therapist's buzz word, but the reality is that having a low opinion of yourself is something that can hold you back in life, make you feel depressed and generally have you wishing you were someone else. Self-esteem is basically all about the way you treat yourself inside, what you say to yourself, how you respect yourself and what you do to meet your own needs. The problem is that most people with low self-esteem have been taught not to look after themselves. The good news is that all is not lost, as it's never too late to find your self-esteem. Here's how:

Teach yourself to feel better

The best way to do this is firstly to hang around people who have good self-esteem. These are the people who feel good about themselves, and their lives. They don't put themselves down, but at the same time they don't go around telling everyone they are gorgeous and fabulous. The way you can spot someone with high self-esteem is to watch how they support others and still have the confidence to ask for help and advice.

Silence the voice in your head

The trick with building your self-esteem is to stop listening to your internal critic and to replace it with a voice that's more supportive. The way to do this is to question what you're saying to yourself. How do you know you can't do it? Why are you protecting yourself? What's the worst that can happen here? What's your real issue wth this problem?

Build a meaningful life

If you can find your niche in life and have a positive appreciation of your achievements you'll naturally feel good. Feeling that you are competent boosts self-esteem – so learn to trust your decisions and not to agonise over what you should have done.

Just be nice to yourself

Yes, it couldn't be simpler than that. Practise being nice to others, and inside your head being nice to yourself, and it will become second nature. Plus, it's easier to think nice things about people than to be forever nasty. Even better, being nice has a follow-on effect of not only boosting your esteem but also activating your brain to push up your happiness quota. After all, it's hard to feel miserable when you're thinking positive thoughts.

Babe pointers

+ **Avoid judgements** Can you accept people without judging them? If not, then you need to look at how harshly you judge yourself. Criticism of others reflects our own levels of insecurity and how we view the person we are inside. If we can't accept others, we can't accept who we are inside.

+ **Get out of your comfort zone** It's always comforting to stay where you are, even if you're unhappy and down on yourself, because you know what to expect and how your life will turn out. However, it always pays to move yourself out of your comfort zone and challenge yourself to change. This is the first step towards better self-esteem.

+ **Give yourself five compliments a day** It sounds easy and it should be, so if you're struggling to find five things it means you definitely need to think more highly of yourself. Things to pat yourself on the back for can include absolutely anything, from 'Today I found three things to compliment myself on instead of two' to working out a problem at work.

+ **Learn to accept compliments** Stuck for something to say when someone throws you a nice comment? Well, all you have to say is 'Thank you'. Turn it down, or shrug it off, and you'll stop getting compliments.

How to be uninhibited

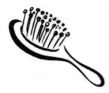

Uninhibited girls know how to have fun, how to let down their hair, how to run screaming around a room, how to embarrass themselves just for the fun of it and generally how to have the time of their lives. The truth is they are no braver, funnier and sillier than we are, they just care less about what others think, and so do more than others do. One major clue that you're too controlled for your own good is your simply not being able to seize the day for fear of what will happen tomorrow. If you wake up with regrets or look back and wish you had simply been sillier, wilder and generally less controlled, here's how to be uninhibited.

Forget about tomorrow

Relax – your world won't fall apart if you just loosen your rules for a day. While it's great to have personal rules, the fact is they are there to structure your life, not hem you in. Are your rules too hard and fast? Do yourself a favour – give yourself a week-long break. For seven days, don't follow your rules.

Let loose

When was the last time you really let your hair down and did something a little crazy? If you can't remember, it's time to jump off that square of security you've been sitting on. Join a tap-dancing class, learn to salsa, take up boxing, go bungee jumping. Do something thrilling, bizarre and generally totally out of the norm for yourself. Regularly pushing yourself out of your comfort zone is essential for uninhibited living. Not only does it build confidence but also it boosts self-esteem and makes you believe you're capable of more than you ever imagined.

Consider the worst that can happen

If you're still stuck with the words 'I can't do that because…' it's worth considering the worst that can happen if you do take that jump into the unknown. Write a list of the downsides and take it to the extreme. Now read your list back and think how much of the 'worst' could actually happen. Would it be so awful if you went to work with a hangover for one day? Would it be so bad if you fell over or danced like a fool, or wore something sexy and not black when you next went out? Remember: our minds tend to protect us from perceived harm, meaning every time someone comes up with an idea we find threatening, our brains will automatically search for get-out clauses.

Be a 'Yes' woman

As in, start saying 'Yes' to things you would have previously said 'No' to. You may feel like a night in on the sofa, but how many times does someone offer you a free ticket to a night on the town, or the chance to meet someone new?

Laugh at yourself

Finally, learn to laugh at yourself. People who are afraid of falling over usually worry not because of the pain factor but because of the potential embarrassment it can cause. The fact is no one ever died of embarrassment, and even if you feel humiliated it's only a momentary thing.

Babe pointers

✦ **Have a consuming passion** Or rather, find one (and boyfriends don't count). Think sporting challenge, music, books, salsa dancing, even cooking – anything is possible, and you'll be amazed at what it brings to your life.

✦ **Take risks** Otherwise known as: try it once before you turn it down. So you've never snorkelled/danced/made a speech – it doesn't mean you can't do it, or will hate it. Many a mad passion has been discovered by accident.

✦ **Don't listen to detractors** The problem with being inhibited is you've probably surrounded yourself with equally inhibited people warning you about the potential pitfalls of doing anything risky or risqué. Don't listen to them, just try and see if it works for you.

✦ **Be bonkers** Just once – it won't kill you!

How to look good in clothes

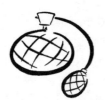 Ever noticed how some people can just walk into a second-hand shop and come out looking as if they've strolled off a catwalk, and others can pick up something cheap and tatty and make it look as if it were a couture outfit? If this is not you, you're not alone. Most of us either are stuck in an era when we felt we looked our best (combat trousers, anyone?), or have a uniform of jeans, T-shirts and trainers that we know we look good in. However, nothing can change your image faster than the clothes you wear, and the rules are simple; here's how to do it.

Search for a new look

Go through fashion magazines and pull out anything that takes your fancy. Choose pictures that reflect whole looks, as well as types of jeans, shirts, dresses and accessories. Avoid focusing on the fact that the clothes are all being worn by models but concentrate on the way they have been put together. You're looking for a style you can copy or make your own.

Try things on

Also known as: don't be afraid to experiment. Clothes on hangers don't always reflect how clothes may look on your body, and colours that you are sure don't suit you sometimes look much better than anticipated. Don't be afraid to take a variety of clothes into the changing room, and make sure not only that you look at yourself in a full-length mirror but also that you have a whole outfit in there with you. While there are no hard-and-fast rules to wearing clothes, it's worth noting that flesh bulging out over low-rise trousers at the front and/or back looks unattractive, as do gaping buttons on a shirt.

Get the perfect fit

Likewise don't be a slave to a dress size. As depressing as it may feel to try on a large when you're convinced you're a small (or want to be), bear in mind that the larger size will be a better fit and therefore make you look longer and leaner. With shirts, always try hugging your arms around your body to check that the shirt is comfortable. Then lift your arms up and if the shirt rides up more than 2.5cm (1in), go up a size. Skirts should literally skirt over your stomach and bottom and not cling, and trousers shouldn't cling at the crotch or the bottom. Likewise avoid going baggy. Large clothes don't hide bulges, but accentuate your size.

Babe pointers

+ **Don't shop in the men's department** You'd be surprised at how many women go down this path, their thinking being that baggier is better. The truth is even a man's small will be too big for most women, as men's clothes are made to fit different dimensions (they have larger shoulders and smaller hips, for a start). It's always better simply to go up a size in your own section.

+ **Mix and match** The key to looking fabulous is to buy one good-quality item and then mix it with a cheaper article of clothing. Good-quality gear should be the long-lasting stuff – coats, shoes and boots. Cheaper items you can get away with include tops, skirts, accessories and jeans.

+ **Wash your clothes properly** Meaning always read the label. If it says 'dry-clean only' – only dry-clean it. Watch what can be dried at high temperatures and what can't, and avoid throwing all your colours into the same wash. All these things help protect your clothes and make them last longer.

+ **Don't follow fashion blindly** Blue eyeshadow, white stilettos and drainpipe jeans may be 'in', but if you have olive skin, short legs or thighs as big as tree trunks, it's probably not a wise move for you. It's fine to take your tips from the fashion pages, but don't go down the copycat route. Dress to suit your own style and body.

How to give advice

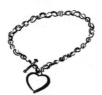

It's just common sense, isn't it? Well, yes, advice is just common sense, but the problem is we all have a different view of what actually makes sense and what doesn't. If you're still determined to be the local agony aunt, here's all you need to know about problem-solving.

Never offer advice unless you're asked for it

Unsolicited advice will go down as fast as the *Titanic*. So no matter if you see disaster racing up at 100 mph, do not offer your 'view' if it hasn't been asked for. Exceptions to this rule include matters that directly affect you, problems of biblical proportions (think hospital, police and a stay in prison) and friends who constantly waste your time by making the same mistake, over and over.

Only say it once

Also known as: save your breath and salvage your friendships. If a friend constantly revisits you with the same old refrain, don't become part of her pattern.

Work out what people want from you

A strange irony exists with advice-giving – not everyone who asks for advice actually wants it. For your own sanity, work out which person genuinely wants your advice and who doesn't.

Be careful how you say things

Tough love isn't always the best option. As tempting as it is to shout, 'PULL YOURSELF TOGETHER,' life is made up of many sensitive souls who need to hear their advice cushioned by something softer.

Censor what you say

The key with advice is not to think about what you would do in the same situation, but to put yourself into the shoes of the problem-seeker and consider what their options are. This means, don't always say what you think, because honesty is subjective.

Don't be their therapist

Contrary to popular belief, giving advice is not the same as counselling. Your job isn't to analyse a friend's soul and discuss what happened to them in childhood.

Don't be afraid to say you don't know

Confused by a dilemma? Worried that they will take your opinion to heart? Simply unsure of what to say? Then don't be afraid to say you don't know.

Don't be upset if they don't take your advice

Asking for advice is like asking for directions. People don't expect you literally to take them to where they want to go; they just need to know a possible route to get there.

You'll never get the whole story

Despite what people say, there are always going to be factors you haven't been told about. So, bear in mind that a large piece of the jigsaw may be missing. If a story feels odd, it probably isn't the whole story – and you should give your advice accordingly.

Babe pointers

✦ **Remember it's their problem not yours** Avoid becoming part of the drama.

✦ **Don't forget your own problems** Resist becoming the person to whom everyone always spills out their problems. Set clear boundaries with people. Remember your life too.

✦ **Avoid taking responsibility for someone else** As tempting as it is to want to help a friend, do not take responsibility for their actions. Give advice, and be clear that this is just one option.

✦ **Let people make their own decisions** They may have taken up all of your Saturday night, but this doesn't mean they have to do what you say. Always bear in mind you are dishing out advice, not dictating a person's actions!

How to stay calm

Staying calm in the modern world is not an easy thing. If it's not road rage, phone rage, boyfriend rage or just plain all-round rage getting you down, it's the general stress and worry of everyday life. Yet staying calm has less to do with meditation, burning incense sticks and not letting life bother you, than knowing what battles to choose. Fight every irritation and you're asking for less calm and more trouble. Here's how to maintain your inner peace.

Think before you act

It may not feel like it but we all have power over our responses, even if they feel automatic. This means that if you consciously act to interrupt your thought pattern, you can stop yourself feeling angry, annoyed and irritated, then instigate calmness in your head. The way to do this is to stop, breathe and then put the situation into perspective before you do anything. Is it the end of the world? Have you been hurt? Will it help to get angry/annoyed/mad? Then rationally consider what emotion will enable you to deal with the situation and give you the outcome you want.

Breathe

When we're stressed and in a state of panic, we tend to take shallower breaths, which hinders proper breathing and stops us thinking clearly. This is why the old counting-to-ten argument can help. By slowly counting you are giving yourself time to breathe, time to calm down and time to think. Try diaphragmatic breathing for optimum results – breathe in and imagine your stomach swelling like a balloon, then breathe out and imagine it deflating; repeat five times.

Don't be a control freak

Even the best-laid plans go wrong at times, so there's no point in falling into a panic if life doesn't go the way you want it to or complaining about the unfairness of it all. Learn to let go of what you can't control, such as other people's behaviour, the weather and so on, and focus on what you can change and deal with, such as your response. Remember: trying to manage others is also a no-no if you're trying to stay calm and composed.

Eat properly

It might seem weird to have this in here, but our bodies work on the fuel we give them. The higher the grade of food, the better your mind and body will function. If you want to feel calm, don't turn to alcohol, tea and coffee, junk food and cigarettes for help. All these stimulants will do is lower your blood-sugar level and cause mood swings and tiredness, as well as boosting anxiety and tension levels. For inner calmness – stay clear of caffeine and sugar, alcohol and nicotine.

Babe pointers

- ✦ **Take a break** Five minutes of daydreaming here and there, a good hearty laughter break and a quick walk can all invigorate you and help you to stay calm in stressful situations.
- ✦ **Drop the 'I should's** They are all the things you feel you ought to do but are just another way to stress you out and make you feel anxious. Give yourself a break; you're doing the best you can, you can't do everything, so don't overtire yourself trying.
- ✦ **Tune people out** It sounds mean, but there are certain people in our lives whom we love, but who stress us out, which is why it can help to tune them out when they're annoying us.
- ✦ **Say 'No' more often** We're all guilty of saying 'Yes' because we're afraid to say 'No', but all this does is cause us to over-commit ourselves and have no space to stay calm and relax.

How to be a domestic goddess

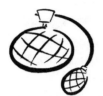 If your knickers and clothes pattern your bedroom and bathroom floors, magazines and papers dated post 1990 pile up by the TV, and unopened mail lies scattered somewhere between toilet rolls and clean laundry – I'm talking about you. Feng-shui experts would say living in a clean and clear environment makes for a clean and clear mind. Whether you believe in this or not, what's true is you'll never feel calm at home if you spend your days stepping over cat-litter trays, kicking pizza boxes under your sofa and wondering if your bath used to be white. Here are some reasons to be clean.

The kitchen

Unseen by our feeble eyes, millions of chomping bugs and mouldy fungi live on our kitchen cleaning equipment. Half-heartedly wipe a cloth over a dirty counter and then throw it in the sink and they celebrate by multiplying. In fact, here's a thought – analysis of over 1,000 kitchen sponges at the University of Arizona found one in five tested positive for salmonella, E. coli and staphylococcus – all food-borne poisonous bacteria, which can make you throw your guts up. All you have to do is buy a new sponge and dishcloth every two weeks and then make sure you pour boiling water over them every day and squeeze out excess water so that they can dry.

The bedroom

A room that is too warm, with no ventilation and in which the pillows, mattresses, blankets and linens are too old and rarely, if ever, cleaned increases your chances of having an allergy. First and foremost wash your sheets every week, at a high (80-degree) temperature, and then use allergy and dust covers on mattresses and pillows before putting the sheets on, although these are next to useless on old pillows and mattresses that are already infested with mites and mite faeces, and their favourite nosh – our dead skin cells. Keep your bedroom well ventilated, as mites thrive on warmth and moisture.

The bathroom

'An enriched Petri dish on a stick' is how experts describe our trusty toothbrushes. And while they make it clear that this isn't a reason to stop brushing our teeth, it's worth noting that the damp bristles you scrub with every night are a perfect breeding ground for bugs, especially flu germs and the herpes virus. Worse still, cockroaches can be attracted at night to the food remnants left on the bristles. Dentists suggest changing your brush every three to four months, but if you've been ill, discard your toothbrush and buy a new one once you feel better (or else you'll re-infect yourself), and store your brush in mouthwash.

Your fridge

Finally, what's lurking in the depths of your refrigerator? If you don't know, it's time to look and then throw out anything that's blue, furry or generally smelly (and shouldn't be). That apart, there are use-by dates on food for a reason. Forget about the waste angle and think about how your stomach and nose will thank you.

Babe pointers

+ **Wash your household stuff as much as your clothes** The same goes for your nice fluffy bath towels: rub yourself vigorously and you'll shed dead skin cells by the bucketload; leave your towel in a damp heap on the floor and the cells will turn mouldy, attracting other bugs to set up home.
+ **Buy new bedding** The Sleep Council advise replacing beds and beddings before they are worn out. Follow guidelines that recommend that a mattress is replaced every eight to ten years and pillows every three to five years (more if a variety of people have slept on them).
+ **Clean once a week** But do a proper all-over clean once a month to get rid of more than surface-level dirt. If all else fails, invest in a cleaner – it might mean one night out less a week, but if your house is clean you may actually want to stay in for a change.

How to survive a hangover

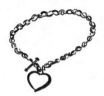

Prevention rather than cure may be the best solution to a hangover, but realistically you are probably not going to go down that path, so here's how to survive that morning-after/going-to-die feeling. First, it's worth noting that all hangovers are not made the same. Although they are obviously all caused by the same thing, the variations on how you feel when you wake up are caused by other factors, such as what you ate (especially at 2.00 a.m.), whether you smoked, how much you shouted when drunk and what you actually did. Whereas it's hard to avoid crossing the line from drunk to drunk and insane, it's worth noting that knowing your danger zone will help you to avoid the grimmer side of feeling bad. Here are some things to remember.

A fry-up is not a cure

The reason hangovers and fry-ups go hand in hand is because fat helps combat the acid lying about in your stomach post drinking, that is, it literally does help you to feel better for a while. Plus, carbohydrates (all that bread you're scoffing) can give you some much-needed energy. However, beware: nothing will have you feeling lethargic faster than this type of food. Fat not only slows down your digestion but also doesn't help the body to metabolise (that is, process) the alcohol in your body. Your aim should be to stabilise your blood sugar (an imbalance being why you feel so hungry and yet so tired), so you need to eat small portions of healthy food frequently. Think about tea, toast, honey and a banana, scrambled eggs and even porridge or cereal.

Hair of the dog is not a cure

Drinking more alcohol the morning after the night before is not a cure for a hangover. Be honest with yourself, it's just a way to tip yourself over into drunkenness again and, therefore, feel better for a short space of time. Water is the only liquid cure you want to drink with a hangover. Also avoid coffee, which will just have the effect of making you feel more dehydrated and painfully aware of all your hangover symptoms. Drink at least 1.5 litres (2 1/2 pints – about eight to ten glasses) of water, plus two extra glasses of water for every alcoholic drink you had last night; or opt for a 250ml (8fl oz) glass of water every 30 minutes.

Don't give yourself a hard time

So you got drunk – it's not the end of the world, even though you might feel as if it is. The fact is the best cure for a hangover is to give in to it, get a blanket, lie down on the sofa and do nothing but drink water. For a killer headache (caused by blood vessels constricting owing to dehydration), take a painkiller. Finally, have a nap – your body will thank you.

Babe pointers

+ **Eat before you party** Your mother was right: a full stomach slows down alcohol absorption and so stops you getting drunk too fast. Good foods to eat are ones that are easily digested so you don't get bloated.
+ **Take a supplement** Milk thistle is a herbal remedy which helps detoxify the liver and improve digestive function, thereby helping you to fight that hangover before it arrives.
+ **Consider your mood** Feeling hyped up or low and blue? Well, it's worth knowing that increased adrenalin helps you to get drunk faster. Hormones also play a vital role, as during ovulation alcohol is absorbed at a faster rate into the body, so watch where you are in your cycle before you start downing double shots.
+ **Take some exercise** Doing a gentle form of exercise, or even having sex, can also help you to sweat the alcohol out, but more importantly both release feelgood chemicals (endorphins) from the brain, which instantly make you feel better.

How to bounce back from any disaster

We're talking resilience here – the ability to jump back and make a rapid recovery from any of life's misfortunes. Whereas we can't stop adversity from happening, research shows that the way we bounce back and deal with nasty setbacks determines our success levels. Let heartbreak, career stagnation, being sacked or having a horrible past crush you and your bounce quota will be low. Stare it in the face with the following tips and you'll not only make it past the hard bits but also sail right on into the sunshine. Here's how.

Work around the problem

Disaster happens: people break up, jobs get cut, and bills arrive with a loud bang on the doormat. Much of dealing with this comes from how aware you were that the crap was about to hit the fan. If you had noticed the signals and prepared yourself, the chances are you'll bounce back far quicker. Pay attention to your life – you won't regret it.

Learn from your experience

The best way to bounce back is to take a look at what went wrong. Break it apart, and see what happened and what you can learn from it. Was it a bad job to start with, the wrong man or a situation that spiralled into disaster? What would you do if you had to do it all again?

Start slowly

Not only because you'll be less likely to make mistakes but also because it's tempting to change too radically after disaster hits. Dating your ex's best friend is not a good idea; neither is changing careers just because you got fired. Likewise, applying for VSO, donating all your clothes to charity and accepting the first offer that comes your way is all bad news.

Note your progress

The good thing about restarting your life and bouncing back is you're likely to see rapid improvement in a short space of time. Be sure to note this down, because sometimes it's hard to see how far you've come. If you've just broken up with someone, note how you were feeling a week ago compared to now. If you were in debt last week, what have you done in the last month to improve the situation? If you're unemployed, how many jobs have you applied for and/or looked for?

Capitalise on your strengths

List all your strengths in a positive way, that is: you're not stubborn, you're tenacious; you're optimistic, not a dreamer; and then look at how you can make them work for you in this situation. Remember: bouncing back has less to do with pure luck and more to do with your attitude. A winning combination is simply to keep on trying even when you feel like giving up.

Babe pointers

✦ **Don't focus on failure** So you lost out/got sacked/had your heart broken – it doesn't have to define you unless you let it. Focus on what you're going to do now, not on replaying how it happened.

✦ **Rethink your goals** An ideal time to regroup and start a new plan is when you're down. Enlist the help of an expert appropriate to your disaster, and then focus on what you now need to accomplish rather than on the ground you've lost.

✦ **Don't go crazy** Tempting as it is to sell up and emigrate or cut all your hair off, don't do it! A change is not always as good as a rest. If in doubt, ask a friend you trust for an honest opinion on your new ideas.

✦ **Figure out if you're shooting yourself in the foot** Especially if disaster keeps happening over and over again, because it's likely you're either repeating the same thing or travelling down the same path without recognising it.

dating

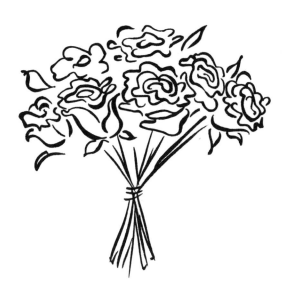

How to catch someone's eye

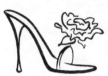 The world of subtle flirting just doesn't hack it when it comes to men. It's not that they're dim (well, hopefully), shy or playing hard to get it, it's simply that most guys have no idea what the heck you're doing and why you're doing it. Mind you, that's not the only point to flirting. While getting a boyfriend on your arm may be your primary objective, knowing how to flirt well is also about knowing how to show others your hidden talents and inner appeal. Do it right and you'll have the power to charm and impress with a simple look. Unsure of how to begin, or just lacking in flirt confidence? Here's how to do it.

You don't have to be gorgeous

Studies show that the power of flirting lies not in how pretty, clever or funny you are, but in the signals you send out. So start by becoming aware of how you respond when men approach.

Giggling, staring blankly and saying 'What?' aren't hot flirt moves. If you're stuck for words (or they are stuck in your throat), don't despair: your flirting moves are registered in your overall demeanour, not your words. Fifty-five per cent comes from your body language (so don't move away, or flinch when he goes to touch your arm), 38 per cent from the way your voice sounds (think friendly tone, voice and attitude) and only 7 per cent from what you actually say (if you're truly stuck, just say 'Hi').

Don't give up before you begin

Constant whining about how you're going to be single for ever and where all the good guys are not only squashes your chances of being flirted with but also will grab the attention only of someone who feels the same way as you do – and who wants to go out with him? Endless studies show the brain believes what we tell it. So tell yourself no one will ever fancy you because you are too fat and ugly and have thighs that meet in the middle, or complain that all the good men are taken and all that's left is rubbish, and you'll never feel like flirting with anyone.

Take a risk (and get up if you are knocked down)

Successful flirts are successful not because they grab more attention but because they take risks and are willing to get up and try again when someone knocks them back. Relive your dating failures over and over and all you're really doing is reliving the rejection.

The best flirt tip in the world: DON'T LOSE YOUR BRAIN!

Flirting, when you get good at it, is addictive, which then makes it something you'll want to do with everyone. However, be selective about who you flirt with. Above all, once you've conquered the initial sequence of getting someone to come to your side, do your best to avoid the trap of self-absorption. If you're too busy worrying what he thinks of you, or what your tummy and/or hair looks like, or even about the next thing you're going to say, it's unlikely you're paying attention to *his* flirt signals. Meaning how are you going to tell if he's interesting and interested in you?

Babe pointers

+ **Flirting is simple** Don't be fooled – it's simpler than you think and any old fool can do it. Look someone in the eye, smile, watch his response and walk over.

+ **Ask open-ended questions** If you are truly stuck for something to say – always ask a question. Remember everyone loves to talk about himself or herself.

+ **Retain a sense of dignity** Yes, you will pull in a low top and micro-mini – but if this is not the 'real' you the question is: who exactly will you attract? Be yourself first.

+ **Always leave him wanting more** Also known as: don't overstay your welcome and make him want to run away from you. Flirt, have fun, get his number and then leave before the lights come up.

How to talk to a man

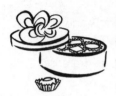 If you're of the belief that women are from Venus and men are from another galaxy altogether, plus find your brain turns to mush the second a good-looking man talks to you, here's what you need to know about talking to men. First, it's not as hard as you think because most men are craving to be spoken to by a friendly woman. Secondly, you don't have to say something witty, smart and intelligent for a man actually to want to talk to you. Whole conversations have been held about something as mundane as a packet of crisps or the state of the wallpaper, and still a relationship has been ignited. If, however, fear strikes you mute here's what you need to do to rev up your conversation engines.

Practise chatting up the postman

Talk to more men. Not men you fancy but men you don't: the postman, the newsagent, the bus conductor, the guy in the café, and the man standing next to you at the photocopier. Chat to them in order to demystify the status you've given men in your brain. The secondary effect of this is it will stop your body from automatically falling into the 'fight or flight' response when a guy talks to you. If fear has rooted you to the spot, think outwards not inwards. He's not looking at the way your hair sticks up at the back, he's waiting for you to speak. Stuck for what to say? Then try asking questions, make a comment about the weather, or say something ridiculous – do anything to help build your confidence around men.

Learn from others

Watch how your friends do it. Noting how other women talk to men can also help. Look for the non-verbal ways they use to make someone feel comfortable: moving towards them as they speak, lightly touching their arm, and smiling. If in doubt always start a conversation with the non-personal, as this makes people feel more comfortable and less like they are being interrogated. And listen, listen, listen … this is what will help you to gauge whether he's interested, what he's interested in and how to respond to the questions he's asking you.

Talk _to_ not _at_

At the other end of the spectrum don't talk _at_ men; constant blathering and not leaving a space for someone to answer your questions is a no-no of the highest order. Things to avoid are: spilling too much information all at once – he doesn't need to know that you loved your first cat more than life itself and how once you were taken to hospital with your head stuck inside a pan. Likewise, don't ask questions that have a preordained answer in your brain. 'How do I look?', 'Notice the difference?', 'Have I gained weight?', and 'Do you like my new haircut?' all fall into this category. Finally, men rarely have opinions on other men's looks, other people's boyfriends and shoes – so save that for your best friends.

Babe pointers

+ **Vary the things you talk about** Make sure you don't make the conversation all about him just to impress him.
+ **Don't let him hijack the conversation** If he's boring you rigid with how 'interesting' his job is and you find yourself nodding off, take control of the conversation by steering it in a different direction.
+ **Keep the conversation going** Use open questions such as 'What do you think of this place?' rather than 'Do you like it here?', which will just get a yes/no response.
+ **Don't be freaked by silences** All conversations have natural pauses, but if the worst comes to the worst and your mind goes blank and you can't think of anything to say, pretend you're interviewing him and go down the who, what, where and when path – it will save you every time.

How to get a man to like you

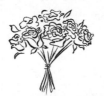

In this age of super-dating it's easy to fall into the trap of thinking there are ways and means to get any guy to be interested in you. The fact remains if he's part interested you can make him more interested, but if he's not at all interested then you're wasting your time, effort and social skills. There is no tried and tested way to get a man to fall for you (despite what certain books say) although there are plenty of ways to get him to like a fake version of you. So here's what not to do and one simple thing to do when manhunting.

Don't be what you think he wants

What do men want? That is the eternal question! Think you've got to be what you think a man wants you to be, and you'll not only lose yourself but also lose him in the process. Being single has a nasty side-effect and it often makes perfectly sane women imagine they are single for a reason. The reality is when a connection is right, it's right. Which means you can have a spot on the end of your nose, say something incredibly stupid and wear knickers the colour of a winter sky and he'll still think you're the sexiest thing he's ever laid eyes on.

Don't be his ex-girlfriend

OK, so he always goes for blondes who like football and do a great show of witty one-liners. Although turning into a shadow of her will work for a while, sooner or later it will get too weird for words, so, basically, don't do it. Far better for your self-esteem, confidence and general happiness to be yourself and let a guy fall for that.

Don't take on his interests

While it's good to be interested in the person you're interested in, make sure you're being honest about what you like. Otherwise you will be the girl asked along to Saturday morning football practice in the rain for the entire season, and you won't have anyone to blame but yourself.

Don't fit the stereotype of the so-called ideal woman

All men want a girlfriend with big boobs, long legs, blonde hair and a flat stomach, a sense of humour, good kitchen skills, great bed skills … the list is endless. Go down it and you'll not only be spending a fortune on plastic surgery, but you'll also be driving your friends bonkers. If you think like this it's time to give yourself a self-esteem check – and repeat the following: you can't second-guess what a man wants and you can't follow an equation for attraction, simply because there isn't one.

To get a man to like you, follow the obvious

Your mum said it, the experts say it and in your heart you know it. Men like women who like themselves! Love your interests, feel cool about the way you look, feel you have something to offer in a relationship, and any man will fall over himself to get you.

Babe pointers

✦ **Be yourself** To get someone to like you, let them get to know the real you. Being mysterious and elusive only works in the movies. In real life, guys want to get to know you and know that you're sincere.

✦ **Stick around** Love at first sight isn't the only way to connect with someone. Build rapport through conversation, sharing, and having a good time, and it will get you to where you want to be.

✦ **Don't tell him your life story (yet)** Always leave him wanting more. Don't lose your value by being too available to his every whim and scheme. Have a life of your own where you have things to do that don't concern him.

✦ **Opposites do attract** But look a bit closer and you'll see that people who look fundamentally different on the outside often have similar objectives and interests. Be honest with yourself – you may fancy the pants off him but what's his long-term potential for you?

How to find Mr Right

Oops, if this is the part where you think I am about to divulge the million-dollar secret to finding your Mr Right or condone the do-anything-to-get-a-man-theory, I'm sorry to disappoint. As shown by the high divorce rate and the many books on the subject there is actually no guaranteed way to find (and keep) Mr Right. Which leads us nicely on to the subject of how to try to find your Mr Right. Here's what you need to know.

Know what you're looking for

Experience shows that the best analogy for finding true love is going shopping for an important event. Essentially, you need to know what you're looking for. If you don't go out with a clear idea of what you want, then you're likely to panic-buy and either come back with something that doesn't fit properly or something that just doesn't suit you. So, basically, know what you want and why and you won't have to throw it all away.

Look in the right places

The above should point you in the right direction in terms of locating Mr Right. If you're a homebody who hates noisy clubs, it's no good doing all your flirting in a bar every weekend. It's also no good desiring an Adonis with a six-pack if the most work your trainers have ever seen is the walk from the fridge to the TV. Studies show that like attracts like. So if you want a sporty person then become a sporty person.

There's more than just one

Consider the question of 'the ONE'. Contrary to romantic mythology, there are lots of 'Ones' for you. Meaning there are plenty of men out there who can play Mr Right fantastically well, and plenty of different men you will be able to live happily ever after with.

What have you got to offer?

If you spend all your time collating information about what you want/need and intend to have from your Mr Right, then you're likely to forget an important part of this equation: what is *he* looking for? Despite the bad rap men get as being visual creatures (and let's be honest here, looks play a big part for all of us), men are also looking for qualities in their partners, and the good news is the qualities tend to be the same as the ones you're looking for. That means they are looking for well-rounded, interesting people – which you won't be if 99 per cent of your time is spent looking for a date, talking about dates and lamenting the state of your dates.

Get out there

Unless you intend to date the gas man or the postman, you need to get off the sofa and venture into the world to find Mr Right. This doesn't mean endless nights in bars but means spreading your net wide. It isn't pathetic to tell people you're looking: go on blind dates, consider the personals and try Internet dating. It isn't sad to ask your friends to set you up, or to go up to a complete stranger and ask him out. If you feel embarrassed or weird about doing any of the above, consider this: if you happen to find an amazing man who makes you blissfully happy, are you really going to care where you met him?

Babe pointers

+ **Timing is everything when it comes to love** We tend to find partners who want the same things as us. So if you're constantly finding men who aren't ready to settle down, consider whether you really are.
+ **Don't be fixated on finding love** Or you'll forget to have a life that you'll be able to share with someone when they do come along.
+ **Be realistic** You're not going to go through the whole of your life without a date or a boyfriend, and if you've gone through a dry spell it's time to shake yourself up and try something new.
+ **Keep your eyes open** Friends have found their Mr Rights in the oddest of places: the local takeaway, on a bus, at the airport, even in the dentist's surgery. This doesn't mean jumping on the first person you meet, but being open to love anytime and anywhere.

How to spot a loser

What's your definition of a loser? A man who wears socks to bed (less of a loser and more of a mummy's boy); a man who at the age of 35 still thinks he's going to be a pop star (deluded rather than a loser); or a boyfriend who names his cars, and his penis, convinces you it's your job to look after his every whim, and then makes sexual passes at all your friends – LOSER, and that's not just him.

The trouble with most losers is they have no idea that they have crossed the line from desirable boyfriend to vile person. The way to lose him is to kick him out. If you haven't already, the real question is: why not?

Those warning signs

If you are someone who thinks she has a loser magnet attached to her forehead and are constantly lamenting how you always get the loser, it's time to get real about who you're dating. The fact is losers always give themselves away. Meaning if you don't spot the warning signals, then you're either too caught up in the idea of having a boyfriend, or being too optimistic about how you can turn them around. Signs to watch out for are:

Men who talk constantly about themselves

Guys who never stop talking about themselves (and it's not first-date nerves) and never ask you a question have high loser potential simply because this indicates a large ego in need of constant massaging.

Men who are attached

This means married, dating, living with someone, separated but still living together, and generally unavailable. Attached guys are a particularly special kind of loser, because they somehow convince themselves they are the good guy and are simply 'misunderstood'.

Men who make passes at other women

These are the men who ogle women's breasts in front of you, try to kiss your friends and then make you feel as if you are a jealous banshee who needs to calm down. While it's not being unfaithful to look and flirt, it *is* being disrespectful and, therefore, is a loud and clear warning sign that the future is not bright.

Men who can't be trusted

This breed of loser tends to give himself away by the second date: he'll either ditch you five minutes before the date begins or forget to turn up, or simply arrive two hours late. This man turns into Mr Unreliable Boyfriend, the guy guaranteed to leave you a bundle of nerves and anxiety wondering if he's going to turn up to your birthday and remember your name.

Men who lie

We all tell the odd little white lie here and there to save someone's feelings, to get out of telling the whole story or generally to entertain others. However, lying sporadically and lying constantly are two very different things. It's the small persistent lies that will give you an indication of the big whoppers to come.

Post diagnosis

How you decide to deal with a loser is up to you, but what you need to ask yourself is not 'Will the love of a good woman change him?' but 'Is this person capable of giving me the love, and relationship, I want?'

Babe pointers

+ **Take off the rose-tinted glasses** While one person's loser is another person's true love, don't delude yourself about someone's true personality traits.
+ **Don't be his therapist** Yes, he may be bordering on the insane because his ex-girlfriend was a loony, and his parents never loved him, but your role is as his girlfriend, not psychiatrist.
+ **Have the same rules for all people** Don't put up with behaviour you would not tolerate in a friend. Make this your benchmark and you won't go wrong.
+ **Don't avoid the signs** Men who let you down consistently, or do things that go against your morals and then laugh it off, are bad news.

How to tell if he's cheating

 Good cheats get away with murder because they are actually schooled in the art of deception. They are the ones who are so used to telling ridiculous little lies that they are desensitised to the bigger ones, and so most of the time forget they are even telling lies. Deluded and deceptive is what we're talking about here and it's tough to catch these men out, as they know the rules of lying.

The good news is the above description doesn't apply to most men. On the whole, if someone is cheating, there are mammoth warnings signs that will ring alarm bells in your head, and a clear path that will lead you right into the lion's den – should you want to venture there. To catch a cheat all you have to do is:

Catalogue what he tells you and why

If you're not a suspicious person and suddenly you're awash with alarming suspicions and find yourself tempted to read his emails, listen to his phone messages and check his neck for perfume that isn't yours, the chances are you've picked up a non-verbal hint that all is not right.

Look at his history

Studies show that men who have been unfaithful to all their partners are likely to do it again. It's not an infidelity gene but a behaviour pattern. Meaning he's addicted to the initial thrill, and the pursuit. If he suddenly falls into patterns that are new to your relationship (but obviously not new to him) – be suspicious.

Body language

There are certain telltale signs when someone is lying or actively good at it. Firstly, born liars often give themselves away by accusing others of lying. A by-product of living in a deceptive way is to assume others are also being deceptive. So if he regularly says he doesn't believe people, watch what he says to you.

Listen to the Chinese whispers

This sounds odd but many an element of truth has been passed on through gossip. That's not to say you should believe everything you hear, but if you've checked out someone's agenda, and then heard something uncomfortable that rings an alarm bell, act on it, if only to dispel your fear.

Consider your alarm bells

We all have a gut reaction for a reason – it's there to warn us about things that are about to fall from a great height on to our heads. If you hear one clanging loudly, don't squash it but consider why it's been triggered. Worried you're being paranoid? Then ask a sane friend to give you her view. If she says your intuition is a measured one then it's time to act on it.

Babe pointers

✦ **Check for give-away signals** Most people are scared when confronted with an accusation of cheating, and so if they then start to lie their auto-nervous system will cause them to sweat more, their breathing will become uneven and they will talk more slowly than usual or get angry really quickly.

✦ **Look for inconsistencies in his story** What parts of the story, if any, don't add up? Is he giving you more information than you asked for – good liars give more details in order to look innocent.

✦ **Don't be fooled by his eyes** It makes no difference whether he's maintaining eye contact or not – some liars can give you a perfectly innocent look and still feed you terrible lies. Trust your gut instinct.

✦ **Think past his answers** What are you going to do if he admits to cheating? Know your two outcomes before you ask him so you aren't stumped for a response either way by his answers.

How to ditch a man

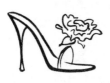 Before going into how to ditch a man, it's worth noting that there is a powerful law of karmic return here. Dump by text, end it with a snippy email, or pretend you've simply dropped off the face of the earth, and you're asking for retribution of biblical proportions. Of course, your method of breaking up depends entirely on the question of why it's over. With non-vengeful break-ups, bear in mind the dignity of the person you're rejecting. Do it in person. And don't tell all your friends before you do it, and/or rub salt into the wound by saying, 'It's not you, it's me,' or suggesting you want to be friends. Instead, try these.

Work out why you're doing it

Like it or not, the 'Why?' question is going to come up, so you had better have an answer on hand, although honesty isn't always the best policy here: you're already breaking up with him – there's no need to kick him when his down.

When to do it

Your birthday, his birthday, Valentine's Day, Christmas Day and the first day of your joint holiday abroad all tend to be very bad days to ditch someone. Likewise, post sex, post a fabulous dinner that he's made, and just after he's introduced you to his family, are also bad times. Do it like that and not only will you pay big time on the guilt front but even your best friends won't be sympathetic to your cause. Ditching someone is all about timing. The ideal time to do it is before a date rather than post meal when he's spent a fortune on you.

Where to do it?

Don't be fooled, a public location will not stop a man going ballistic, crying or attacking you with a fork. This is because his mind will not be fixated on what others are thinking, but simply on the fact you've just broken up with him. For his dignity (and yours) it's better to break up at his place where ranting and begging can be kept between the two of you.

What to say

Less is always more when ditching because no matter what you say there will be a follow-up conversation; meaning don't give out ammunition he can later hit you over the head with. Babble incoherently, say, 'Let's have a break for a while,' and mumble on about things just not being right and you'll be talking about it all night/week/year.

Allow him a response

In an ideal world, we'd ditch someone and they'd proudly maintain a stiff upper lip, shake our hand and go on their way. Reality check: breaking up is about as smooth as rocky-road ice cream. First, he's allowed to make a response, and this is likely to be loud, accusing and maybe even rude (although you don't have to stand there listening to it). Secondly, you will feel guilty – even if he deserves to be dumped and you know you're right. Thirdly, you'll probably cry. Whoever told you it's easier to be the dumper than the dumpee was lying.

Babe pointers

+ **Keep to the point** Listing an itinerary of all the many things he did wrong will only swing you off the point.
+ **Leave him alone post dumping** It's fine to send a text saying, 'How are you doing?', but calling him three times a day because you feel guilty just gives him false hope.
+ **Don't imagine you'll get over it faster than he will** Some guys are happily back out there looking the night after being ditched.
+ **Don't rub his face in it** Preserve his dignity, keep the break-up story to the bare facts.

How to get over being dumped

Getting over a relationship depends primarily on how and why you broke up. Being ditched for a younger model, your best friend, via text or on live TV tends to call for a significantly higher dose of break-up help than simply forgetting to call each other for five months and then waking up one day and realising it's over. How long it takes you depends primarily on what you're getting over. Missing the hot sex and the fact he did all the washing-up is more easily solved than missing the person you're hopelessly in love with.

Of course, part of the problem is that being ditched, dropped, rejected, thrown on the dumper – call it what you may – brings to the surface a number of agonising emotions. First – let's be honest – it hurts like hell. Secondly, the shock often leads to an intense loss of dignity. Think hysterical crying, begging and wailing, 'Pleeease ... don't leave me!' The good news is, this hysteria doesn't last, as long as you pick yourself off the floor and put yourself firmly on the road to recovery.

Call in the cavalry

These are the people in your life designed to offer you the strongest support in times of trouble. Usually best friends, siblings and mothers, all of whom will think nothing of moving in, wiping your snotty nose, telling you he's an idiot and hearing your break-up story told over and over and over. After three days, keep your break-up story to the highlights. This is essential not only for safeguarding your reputation but also because every time you tell the story of being dumped, your brain will trigger all the pain you experienced when it first happened.

Initiate distraction techniques

This works big-time in a break-up because it makes your brain engage in other pursuits besides the urge to call him and beg him to come back. Excellent distractions include exercise, which not only takes your mind off everything besides the fact your body's in physical pain, but also will give you a body that really will make him sorry he left. Bad distractions include food (piling on the pounds won't help your flagging self-esteem), alcohol and home movies of your happier time together.

Get yourself a new life

A change is as good as rest when you're getting over a broken heart, but this doesn't mean cut all your hair off and dig latrines in Africa (this really will not make you feel better). It means take a long hard look at your life and make yourself a priority.

Get angry

It's OK to be mad: he ditched you and left you feeling abandoned – therefore, it's normal to feel furious with him. What's not normal is to pretend he's coming back, delude yourself that you're fine and suggest to him that you should be friends (don't kid yourself: it's impossible to be friends with someone you simultaneously want to kiss and kill). So as the experts say, own your fury and get over him.

Babe pointers

✦ **Accept all offers of help in whatever form they come** Also known as: don't be proud, we've all been there and want to help.

✦ **Revenge isn't sweet** Flirting with his friends, standing outside his house in the pouring rain and sending naked pictures of him to his workmates will only make him wonder why he didn't dump you earlier.

✦ **Don't kick yourself when you're down** Telling yourself he dumped you because your thighs are too big/your boobs too small/because you're needy isn't going to help you feel better.

✦ **Tell yourself this is going to pass because it will** The killer part of a break-up is the mind-numbing mundanity of it all. The waking up and thinking of him, the going to sleep and thinking of him, the waves of nostalgia, the songs on the radio – it's all so endless but it really does end.

How not to be bitter

Dating a horde of losers, watching your friends end up with the men of their dreams and having your heart broken by Mr Right again and again and again are just some of the pills that can turn even the nicest girl towards vengeful and bitter thoughts. If you find bitterness is seeping into your life, here's how to not poison your life.

Avoid all thoughts of ex revenge

Contrary to popular belief, the best cure for heartbreak is not revenge. So do not post his naked butt all over his work website, cut up his clothes and email his mother a list of his worst sexual habits. While all these things will give you momentary satisfaction and large doses of spiteful glee, in the long run they'll leave you still feeling empty and lost. This is because inflicting pain on someone who has caused you pain, ironically, doesn't lessen your pain in any way whatsoever.

Avoid being eaten up by jealousy

Don't feel bitter that everyone else is not suffering like you. If you feel sick with jealousy when you see what others have, remember: they are not loved up and gloriously happy to annoy you, it's just the way it is. Plus, just because they have found happiness doesn't mean they have somehow taken it away from you. Your turn may be just around the corner.

Don't wallow in it

Misery is addictive, as is feeling sorry for yourself, bad-mouthing the world and wearing your PJs all day. As tempting as it is and no matter what has happened, resist the urge to turn your misery into something 'special' that no one understands. Keep telling yourself that you are alone, and that no one else has ever been through your pain, and you will feel alone and go through it on your own.

Life isn't fair

Yes, it's not fair that you've been ditched, but just because you're a good person who has paid her dues doesn't mean that you are owed a handsome boyfriend, ample riches and the best job in the world. Thinking being good should equal a good life is a road to disappointment. Life doesn't work on a point system like this, and you may be the best person in the world and still have to deal with difficult and hard things.

Avoid the bitter pill

Finally, when all else fails and being bitter is the only thing that gets you by, remember it does practically zilch for your looks. Think thin cat-bottom lips, mean eyes and basically no man coming near you for fear of being lashed by your tongue. It's an unhappy state of affairs, so avoid the bitter pill at all costs.

Babe pointers

- ✦ **Get a fantastic life** (hopefully one that will turn him green with envy). The best anti-bitterness solution is to go out and live your life and be happy. Do it properly and he'll be eternally sorry he left you.
- ✦ **Enjoy your jealousy but don't let it drive you down** You can of course have moments of jealousy and despair – you wouldn't be human if you didn't. Just don't let them take over your life.
- ✦ **Make a decision to change** When feeling steeped in bitterness, just make a decision to change. Yes, it is that easy – experts say all you need to do is give your life a major shake-up, make plans, take on challenges and do something.
- ✦ **Choose your friends well** Be careful who you hang around with – bitterness is contagious. Write a list of people who inspire and encourage you, and cull the rest.
- ✦ **Live the life you want** It's hard to be bitter when you're having the time of your life.

How to keep a relationship

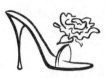 You've waited months, maybe even years, to get to the state of coupledom you're now in. Time for hot nights in together, Sunday mornings reading the paper in bed, long country walks and late-night chats. This is also the time you're most likely to revel in each other, but one day soon Mr Perfect will not be all that perfect – what can save you now? Thankfully the following.

Get some space

As tempting as it is to be a couple of relationship bores, nothing will kill your love faster than spending every night in with a curry and a DVD. You like each other because spending time together is special and it won't be if you're in each other's pockets 24/7. Remember who you are, and surgically remove yourself from his side.

Strap down your needy side

It's OK to need someone and it's OK to be needy; what's not OK is to need reassurance all the time. It's dull for the person you're with and debilitating for you. The truth no one ever tells you is that while falling in love has its wonderful parts, it is also full of dark moments of fear and misgivings. The good news is that this needy stage passes and as you get used to being in love the good then overtakes the bad.

Stop wanting too much, too soon

Slow down – and you know what I mean. If you've already named your children and planned your wedding you need to take a deep breath and think about how long you've been dating. Wanting more is fine, wanting more and pushing for it too early isn't.

Don't try to change him

Likewise, now you've taken off the rose-tinted glasses and can see his flaws, beware of trying to change him. There's nothing more insulting than suggesting a change of career, a haircut and new clothing all in one go. Remember you fell in love with him for who he was, so why are you trying to change him now?

Don't live in each other's pockets

What happened to that life you used to love before you met Mr Right? Where are your friends, your interests, and your career? Why have you decided none of that matters any more? Give up your life for someone and you're guaranteed to feel needy and scared all the time because, basically, without him you will have nothing. Which is why studies show that couples who stay together don't always play together.

Work at it

Finally, having to work at making it work isn't a sign your relationship is wrong but a sign you don't take each other for granted. No matter how long you've been together it always pays to do things that make him happy. At the same time be sure to let him know what he does that makes you happy so he can do more of it; and because it will make him feel appreciated.

Babe pointers

✦ **Don't be smug about being in love**
Your friends will hate you and won't be there to help celebrate your relationship, bear witness to your good times, or mop up your tears when you have a fight.

✦ **When you fight don't overreact**
Everyone argues, it's normal, it's healthy and it's not the end of the world, so do yourself a favour and don't include the whole world in your battles – you'll regret it.

✦ **Don't stop seeing him as a person**
He's not just your boyfriend and partner, he's also someone's son, friend and colleague. Let him play his other roles, too.

✦ **Don't lose your brain or your life**
You had a point of view and a life of your own when you were single, so don't turn into the simpering girlfriend with no mind.

sex

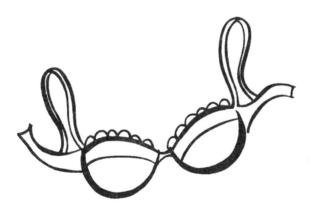

How to talk about difficult sex problems

 We've all heard the spiel: women are from Venus and men are from God knows where. Which is why studies show that communication between the sexes is such a hit-and-miss affair, especially over sex. Wish you could get him to give you more oral, make you climax faster, touch you softer, kiss you longer? Well, you need to learn how to speak his language and get him to interpret yours. Here's how to improve your technique without losing your mind.

Get him to head south

There are many reasons why a man says he won't go down on a woman. Reasons such as 'It's dark and scary' and the strange 'It feels odd'! The truth is most guys who steer clear of oral sex do so because they're scared of doing it wrong and for no other reason. Which means if

you want your guy to go down on you, the best way to do it is to tell him why and exactly how you like it. This will work immediately because: (1) there's no way he'll be able to misinterpret your request; and (2) your A–Z directions will equal a spot-on delivery. Include as many visual descriptions as you can, as this is how guys 'hear' things, and make sure you include the fact that you need a consistent and regular rhythm, a gentle, not rough, pressure and stimulation right through to orgasm.

He's a thruster

If your man's all thrust and no lift-off, then you're not alone. Many men have the bizarre notion that women love vigorous amounts of thrusting, because they don't understand the make-up of the female anatomy. As we know, the part of our body that is the most sexually sensitive is the clitoris and that gets no hit whatsoever from thrusting. If your boyfriend doesn't understand this, and you're raw from waiting for him to come, try highlighting his wrongdoings by showing him the power of a simple clitoral touch. At the same time, try swapping positions. Woman on top will have you controlling the pace and speed – meaning he won't be able to go for a marathon thrust session, and you'll be able to make both of you come faster.

You're a faker

Most men have no idea what a real orgasm looks like so if you're secretly hoping he'll notice, think again. The real question to ask yourself is: why aren't you being honest? Whatever your reason, you need to let him know that your current sex life isn't working for you. The best way to do this is by telling him all the things he does right as this will make him feel confident to try new things. The aim is to make him realise what turns you on, and the best way to communicate this is by show and tell: show him how you like to be touched, and then tell him with loud moans and groans how it feels.

Babe pointers

✦ **Keep sex interesting for your sake and his** Studies show that being proactive during sex equals a more satisfying sex life, more orgasms and a relationship that lasts longer than most. So don't be afraid to initiate new moves and even be the one to kickstart a new sexual idea.

✦ **Actions speak louder than words** If you can't tell him what you want, take control, jump on top, roll him over, grab his hands and place them exactly where you want them to be.

✦ **Talk about sex** Not just about the hard stuff but about the good stuff too. If you can get used to voicing your opinions about your sex life, you won't feel embarrassed when a trickier sexual subject comes up.

✦ **Choose your sex-chat times wisely** Post sex, when half-naked and when you're both tired and fed up are not good 'sex chat' times. Instead, pick a time when you're both relaxed and getting on with each other, and remember: talk, don't criticise, if you want to get somewhere fast.

How to make him a foreplay genius

 If an Indian takeaway is your man's idea of warming up for sex, it's likely his foreplay is about as powerful as an AA battery. With sex studies showing we need at least 20 pre-penetration minutes to rev our orgasm engines, it pays tenfold to improve his foreplay fumbles. The good news is it doesn't take long to teach a man how to perform excellent foreplay. Here's how to teach him to administer some teasing touches.

Indulge in lots of kissing

Studies show that couples who kiss a lot, stay together longer and have better sex. Unsurprising really, as kissing is one of the most intimate and loving things you can do. Make a pact to kiss for five minutes (at least) before you do anything else to each other. Flirt with your lips. Graze his with yours and slowly lick his lips with the tip of your tongue and then blow on them to give him a hot/cold sensation.

Next, while you're indulging in lip-on-lip contact, slowly suck on his lower lip (men love this because the skin is thicker here and it feels sexier). Finally, try moaning while you're kissing, the vibrations will rocket through his body. Now move beyond the lips to other areas of the face. Potential hot spots are his earlobes and ears (though not everyone relishes the thought of an ear bath, so beware).

Teach him to touch you

Unless he's had a fabulous previous girlfriend, he'll be under the illusion that he can treat you like a car: stick the key in and take you from 0 to 60 mph in two seconds. Show him he's wrong by taking him on a tour of your body with a sexy massage. This is not about ironing out his tight muscles in preparation for the 'real thing' but about building your sexual excitement to razor-sharp levels. Take the massage in turns and start by warming your hands with some oil or body lotion. Start by stroking your hands up and down each other's backs, skimming over the bottom and along the sides (the aim is to hit all the erogenous zones in one sweeping movement). Focus on the bum. Go for the small dent above the crease of the bum as this area causes all kinds of tasty ripples when massaged in a circular motion.

Extend the inevitable

Help keep the foreplay mood going by enhancing your staying power and his by both of you exercising your PC muscle (the one that controls the flow of urine). Strengthening this muscle will not only make him last longer but also give you both more satisfying orgasms.

To keep him in the game, the trick is for him to flex/squeeze this muscle when he feels close to the point of no return. This will extend his staying power and boost his thrusting potential. Finally, to boost your orgasm potential, tighten and relax your PC ten times, holding for four seconds each time as you kiss and stroke your way around his body.

Babe pointers

✦ **Remind him that all sex starts in the brain** From that wobble of desire in your tummy, to mind-blowing orgasms – it all begins in your head. Meaning the more powerful your sexual anticipation (and his), the hotter the sex will be.

✦ **Everything counts** Sex doesn't begin only when you take your clothes off, which means everything counts when it comes to foreplay, even your daily emails and texts. Want to get him revved up all day? Then spice up your messages and keep him guessing.

✦ **Take your time** Tempting as it is to rush over the finish line, take your time with your foreplay moves, too. Imagine you're doing a final body check and scrutinise his body. Tease the soles of his feet and the spaces between the toes, and stroke his calves, as these have a super-strong connection to the crotch.

How to turn him on

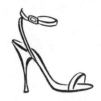

You may have a lover who is the sexual equivalent of the couch potato, but the good news is you can get a response out of him very easily. Countless studies show that men are uncontrollably aroused by sexy sights, meaning give him something to look at and desire and you'll be laughing all the way to bed; the scientific idea being that men are more visually orientated by a sexy image than by a sexy sound or smell. A simple glimpse at your cleavage, a peek at the top of your legs and an eyeful of something naughty will all make him pure putty in your hands. Here's how to make it happen.

Connect with your inner sex goddess

Not some kind of New Age chanting ceremony but more a wake-up call to your inner sexiness. After all, it's hard to act sexy when you don't feel sexy. If you feel self-conscious about parading around in sexy gear, or giving him naughty come-closer looks, you need to learn how to feel sexy about yourself. There is a multitude of ways to do this: step one is to get used to seeing yourself as a sexy person. Start by getting naked more often. Look at yourself in the mirror when you get up and/or out of the bath. Then sit around in the nude and generally get in touch with how your body looks.

Work out how you feel

As in, literally knowing what makes you feel sexy helps you to be sexy. Start off experimenting with underwear, fabrics, smells and even creams. Pamper your body and you'll eventually want to show it off. Next, get physical with yourself. You'll never know what your man can do for you if you don't know what you can do for yourself. Take time out to find out how your body responds to different touches, feelings and sensations.

Love your body

And he will too – simple but true. Women who feel and act as if their bodies are flawed tend not to let go in bed. Keep telling him your tummy is too big and your thighs are too wobbly and that's all he'll start looking at. Instead, throw your shoulders back and prominently display your body. Walk around naked – let him look at you. If you feel too exposed, slip on a sheer shirt, a thin slip and/or even his T-shirt.

Put on a show

Make it seem casual and offhand and he'll love it even more. To pump up his viewing pleasure walk across the room half-naked when you're getting dressed, talk about the weather when you're changing bras and stroking moisturiser up your leg. To really find your sexual groove, put on some music. Nothing will help you lose your inhibitions and find your pace in the bedroom faster than a sexy song.

Babe pointers

+ **Draw his eyes to where you choose** Eyes follow movement, so if you're sitting around having a chat, pull his eyes to where you want. A finger drawn across the collarbone and down the neck draws his eyes to your breasts. Rubbing your ankle pulls his eyes to your legs, and licking and biting your lips means 'Get over here right now'!

+ **Deprive him of visual thrills** Despite the virtues of visual pleasure, sometimes depriving your man of thrills will intensify his other senses and turn up his turn-on quota. Blindfold him in bed and then work on his sense of touch and smell.

+ **Ask him what he likes** This one works every time and will stop you second-guessing. Don't be freaked out if it's the obvious stuff like stockings and heels – it might not be original, but that's not the point.

+ **Tell him how he's making you feel** Men like to know they are doing the right thing, so moan, sigh and basically tell him exactly how it feels.

How to leave him breathless in bed

 Breathless sex doesn't just have to be of the energetic, aerobic kind (although that works, too). If your idea of breathless is basically to surprise him, then you've come to the right place. Here are the most breathtaking things you can do in bed.

Tie him up

According to the world-famous Kinsey Sex Report, 26 per cent of people are aroused by mild bondage activities, so if you've ever fantasised about being tied up, spanked and/or blindfolded, here's your chance to give it a go.

The thrill comes from creating a sense of both anxiety and arousal. Bondage also teaches even the shyest of lovers to be a bit more creative, and the most controlling of people to let go. As the whole point of doing the tying up is so you can play-act at being punishing and controlling, you need to maintain the game. If he speaks or tells you what to do, punish him by stopping what you're doing. He must know you're in charge of his enjoyment and ultimate satisfaction – he has to obey you, as this will heighten his orgasm potential and have him begging for more. However, always be aware of the basics:

1. Never tie anything that restricts breathing.
2. It is always best to decide how far you will go before you start.
3. Choose a word or phrase that you can use that will make you or your partner stop immediately.
4. Keep your bedroom door locked, unless you like the thrill of being caught by your relatives.

Dress up

Whereas fetishism conjures up images of leather-bound people in dodgy nightclubs, the truth is we all have private fixations that arouse us in a sexual way. Think stilettos, stockings, leather, or even tight jeans and a white T-shirt. And don't be fooled into thinking this is just a male thing. There's many a woman turned on by the shape of someone's bicep, leg muscle or hairline.

Have a quickie

Contrary to popular belief, sex isn't always better when it lasts a long time. In fact, there's a lot to be said for 'slipping it under the wire' and having quick, frenzied sex somewhere you're not meant to be. To take his breath away, have fast sex in places where he'd never imagine you would give it a try: a moving train, an alleyway, his parents' bathroom, your office meeting room, or even up against the family Christmas tree. The more illicit you can be, the more tantalising the effect and the more breathless he'll be.

Talk dirty

But be careful, because one person's naughtiness is another person's insult. The reality is most people thrive on a bit of smutty talk, as it adds a small thrill to the event. If you want to give it a try, start having sex and at a crucial bit, say something downright rude. If he speeds up, looks a bit shocked but seems to be turned on, turn it up and go for it.

Babe pointers

✦ **Breathless sex isn't scary sex** By all means push back your sexual boundaries, but go slow and watch his response as you do it. Wide eyes and an open-mouthed look is good; wide eyes and colour draining from his face isn't.

✦ **Do what you want to do** Sexy is as sexy does, meaning if you're into whatever you're proposing, you're going to put more effort in and appear 100 times sexier. Raid your fantasy locker and instigate what will leave you breathless.

✦ **Listen to his hints** Stuck for ideas? Then have a listen to what he's been saying. Did he 'joke' about getting a porn film, tease you about cheap red undies? What makes him flustered? These are your breathless keys.

✦ **When all else fails …** Ask him what he'd like, and tell him what you're hoping for. It sounds contrived but it's guaranteed to work every time.

How to orgasm

The good news is that even if you've never ever had an orgasm, you do have it in you to get there. If you don't believe this, the likelihood is you've either had the wrong lovers or been looking too hard for your big 'O'. The main reason why most women don't orgasm through sex is a simple design fault. Most female orgasms depend on clitoral stimulation. However, the route to male orgasm bypasses the clitoris. Also, studies show that there is a gap of about 17 minutes between the time it takes for a man to reach orgasm and how long it takes a woman – he can get there in three minutes while you'll need 20. Meaning you may just be heading out of the starting gate as he gallops over the finish line. Here's how to get in sync.

All orgasms vary

Waiting for that moment when you scream the house down? Well you may have to keep waiting. The first rule of orgasms is to note that all orgasms vary. Not only from day to day, but from sensation to sensation, and from boyfriend to boyfriend. So do yourself a favour and ignore tales of couples screaming the house down and focus on what you can do to get your excitement levels up. The key here is to work on what gets you going before you work on him.

Bring yourself to arousal and plateau

The body and mind are linked when it comes to orgasm, which is why all the best moves in the world won't work if you're lying back and thinking about the laundry. To help yourself, concentrate on physical stimuli, such as foreplay, oral sex, kissing, stroking each other, and clitoral stimulation, as well as fantasies. Keep adding to the images in your mind while focusing on what you're doing to him and what he's doing to you.

Remember: if the stimulation stops, you will go right back to the beginning and your boyfriend will have to start over.

The orgasm

This is the peak of arousal – if nothing stops you here, you'll be free to pant your way to happiness through a succession of involuntary genital contractions that should last anywhere from ten to 60 seconds, or longer. However, don't get caught up on the type of orgasm to have. Despite talk of simultaneous, multiple and g-spot orgasms, any orgasm is good. If anything, studies show that fewer than 30 per cent of women experience multiple orgasms or simultaneous ones (because of the time lag mentioned above). If you're keen to have more than one orgasm during sex, just go for one during foreplay, another during sex and/or oral sex, and so on. If you can never find more than one, don't feel disappointed – like everything in life it is quality not quantity that counts in the end.

Babe pointers

+ **Learn to do it on your own** Apart from feeling good, this is a guaranteed way to improve your sex life. Know what moves work for you on your own and you can bring them into your sex life and make them work for you when you're together. The keys are an active mind, a relaxed atmosphere and less trying.
+ **Don't be orgasm-obsessed** The reality is orgasms don't happen all the time so don't be disappointed if it doesn't happen. Spend your time obsessing and all that will happen is you'll ruin your sex life.
+ **Think time of the month** Your hormones can affect your orgasm potential more than you think. Around ovulation and prior to your period your chances of having an orgasm are higher, simply because your sex drive is at a peak. Use this to your advantage.
+ **Have more sex** The reality is the more you get to know someone, the higher your chances of having an orgasm.

How to come together

Have you ever noticed how in the movies couples have simultaneous and satisfying orgasms at the click of their fingers? Sadly, as you probably already know, real-life sex isn't so easy. Studies show the chance of reaching peak at the same time as your bloke is fairly low, especially if your bodies are very different sizes and you don't know each other's sex patterns very well. The main problem is that women take longer to build to the pre-orgasmic phase, so when you're both in the same race he'll be over the finish line drinking champagne while you're still warming up. However, the simultaneous 'O' can be done, and here's how.

Arousal is the key

The first trick is to get your sexual responses in sync, which means getting to the same level of arousal. As one slight flick of the hand will probably get him from 0 to 100 in two seconds, so the aim of his game is to delay penetration and ejaculation for as long as possible. The best way to do this is to get him to indulge in mass foreplay on your body, and not to touch him. Studies show that a woman if stroked in the right way will start to become aroused within 30 seconds of being touched, so he won't have to go at it for long. Aim for the erogenous zones: the breasts, the thighs and the genitals.

Plateau stage

To sustain arousal, make sure your guy keeps up his end of the bargain and works on physical stimulation (remember, you can help him out if he gets tired). Warning: if he stops now, you won't achieve any type of orgasm, never mind a simultaneous one. Also, have a swift look at him. If at any stage you see the head of his penis enlarge and his testes draw closer to the body, give up your chances of a mutual climax and go for penetration because he's about to come. If he can hold off, look for signs that you're approaching orgasm so you're ready to make for the next stage. Signs you're close are: the clitoris retracting slightly; a sex flush (a slight reddening) appearing across the breasts and genitals; your heartbeat speeding up; and a deep ballooning feeling deep inside your vagina. Your muscles will also start to tense all over your body, and lubrication will increase. If you can feel all this – you're ready for the finale.

Orgasm

The second your pelvic muscles start to tense up, get your bloke in place and go for penetration. The aim is now to get your pace in sync, so thrust up as he thrusts down. Also, if he lies higher up your body, his pelvic bone will rub the clitoris as he thrusts. If you can build from here at a mutual pace, the likelihood that you'll finally come together is pretty much assured.

Babe pointers

✦ **Don't despair if it doesn't happen** If you try this technique and it doesn't work, don't despair. Mutual climaxing doesn't make for better sex, so relax and focus on having a good time instead. After all, that's the real point of sex.

✦ **Orgasms vary all the time** Orgasms, like most things in life, depend on your mood and the way you go about getting them. Meaning each time will be different for you. So if you want massive contractions each time, the only way to do it is to note what makes you come, but remember: don't write off the little ones – an orgasm is an orgasm whether is a gentle 'Aaah!' or a rip-roaring 'OHHH!'

✦ **There's only one way to orgasm** Reality check: there are at least six different types of female orgasm – clitoral, vaginal, g-spot, multiple, simultaneous and fantasy (on your own), all of which bring different results. So if you can't reach one, try another.

How not to be stressed about your body

If the thought of getting naked and having sex is making your brain send out panicky SOS signals, here are a few tips to help you get a grip. The good news is that anyone and everyone can excel between and outside the sheets. We only imagine we can't because we watch too many fabricated sex scenes on TV. If you want to stop having sex with your stomach pulled in, your clothes half-on and the lights off, here's how to shed your body fears and get over the fear of being naked.

Relax about the naked thing

We all know the feeling: he goes for your clothes, and you go for the light; he suggests a spot of outdoor exhibitionism, and you run for the bushes; he polishes up the mirror, and you turn your back on it. No, you're not shy – more like you hate your body. To help yourself, get used to seeing yourself naked. Women who hate their bodies rarely look at themselves naked. Next, remember: clothes hide only so much. OK, so you think you've performed miracles and made yourself look like a teeny-weeny supermodel, but the truth is, if you're really a medium/large, then that's what he sees, clothes on or not. Which means he fancies you the way you really look, not the way you think he sees you.

Don't compare yourself to his ex

Or any number of celebrities. Unless you have the physique of a supermodel, then it's quite likely that there's something about your body parts that you just don't like. Realise that everyone (even men) worries that their body's not ravishing enough, their technique not expert enough, or their bits not big/small/firm enough. If you think like this – stop (and yes it is that easy, you just focus on something else) because if you can't accept your body the way it is, then how can you expect someone else to?

Focus on your positive points (and yes we all have at least one)

So you hate your stomach? I'll bet you a million pounds he's not even noticed it. Next, be realistic – is all your self-worth really wrapped up in the size of your bra? Finally, think about what you're doing to your boyfriend. No one wants to reassure someone all the time. It's insulting, not to mention exhausting; this man is here not to boost your self-esteem, but to be your lover.

Do something about it

If you really can't bear your naked form, and you're 100 per cent sure it's not all in your mind, then do yourself a favour and do something about it. Not because you have to, but because gaining body confidence boosts sexual confidence and self-esteem. It will not only make you feel better about yourself but also help you to see that it's not how you look but how you feel that counts.

Babe pointers

✦ **Be sensitive about his body too** Men have the same insecurities as we do: most worry they are too fat/thin and that their bodies don't live up to ideal images of washboard stomachs and killer biceps. Meaning be careful how you comment on his body when he's naked.

✦ **You're more than your bust size** And your weight, and your legs, and the size of your stomach; something you won't realise if 90 per cent of your thoughts are based around how unattractive you think you are. Too hung up on how you look? Then practise looking outwards, not inwards.

✦ **Don't be oversensitive** Fretting over one of his throwaway comments? Annoyed that he suggested you get fit together? It doesn't mean a thing if he's still loved up on you, unless of course you make it into a larger than average issue. Remember: actions always speak louder than words.

How to deal with a crap lover

There are many definitions of a crap lover, the primary one being the man who doesn't try, closely followed by the man who thinks he doesn't have to try and then the man you wish would try less. Of course, when it comes to love and relationships, sex isn't everything but, sadly, when sex is bad, sex becomes everything in a relationship. If your sex life has you closing your eyes and thinking of England, here's how to deal with it.

The selfish lover

First up we have the selfish lover: the man who thinks just because he's getting his rocks off and he's OK, so are you. After all, his pleasure is your pleasure, isn't it? Lie back and say nothing and this is the life you have to look forward to. Sadly, the only way to deal with a selfish lover (apart from dumping him) is to yell, 'WHAT ABOUT ME?' in his ear.

Honesty is the best policy here because this is what will pay dividends in the end. If your message goes in one ear and out the other, it means he is genuinely not interested in your pleasure, so why are you getting naked with him?

The oversensitive lover

This is the man who can't bear criticism, the man who responds well when you're singing his praises but can't bear to hear you say the words, 'It might be better if …' Like the selfish lover, this man is more concerned with his ego than with your sexual pleasure, so honesty is the best policy once again. Cushion your words with flattery and he'll be putty in your hands. Tell him it feels fabulous when he does X, but it would feel even better if he did X and Y and then moved swiftly on to Z. Be sure to applaud his moves, and you'll score a 10/10 every time.

The lazy lover

Out of all the worst lovers, this man's the least of your problems because it *is* possible to get him moving. To speed him up and make him try harder, let him know that: (1) you expect much, much more; and (2) you expect it from him. Often lack of guts in bed has a lot to do with a lack of confidence, so tell him you love his moves but wish that he'd use more of them – and watch him move.

The know-it-all lover

This is the man who, when you voice an opinion, says, 'But my exes never complained ...', the man who assumes that when it comes to sex he is 'the' man. Sadly, it's hard to burst his sexual bubble because he'll just assume it's you, not him, but you can reap the benefits by turning the tables on him. Less flattery and more action are the answer in this power struggle. Move your body away if you don't like what he's doing, and move closer when you do, and he'll get the message fast.

Babe pointers

+ **Speak up for what you want**
Despite what you might think, nice girls do like and love sex – so speak up if things aren't right and do something about it (besides grumbling to your mates behind his back).
+ **Men aren't psychic** Especially when it comes to sex. If he's doing something wrong or you want more of something else – don't expect him to: (1) notice; (2) pick up on your subtle hints; and (3) read your mind.
+ **Don't rush it** Good sex takes time and effort, and isn't something that happens instantaneously. Give your sexual relationship a chance to improve before you call it a day.
+ **If all else fails dump him** Having a boyfriend who's inexperienced is one thing, but having a lover who just won't try to change his ways is another. If you've reached a stalemate and he doesn't care, ditch him for someone who will.

How to get to grips with morning-after etiquette

The morning after the night before is a minefield of potential disasters. Should you make him breakfast just because he stayed the night? Can you ask him to leave before 7.00 a.m.? Will he be offended if you admit you've forgotten his name? Shame, awkwardness and hazardous exploits like these all await you, especially if you don't know the right etiquette. To find out how to avoid crippling morning-after embarrassment and how to eject the snoring lump beside you, read on.

How to get rid of a one-night stand

It's simpler than you think: call him a cab. If he says he doesn't want one, give him directions for the bus stop, while passing him his clothes. The aim here is to let him know you want him to leave.

Yes, it feels rude, but what's better: having him stick around because you don't want to offend him or having him leave? If he tries the 'Goodness, I'm hungry' line, point out how close McDonald's is to the train station, and if all else fails, tell him you're leaving too, and head out the door with him (even if it's just to walk around the block).

How to wake up with a potential new boyfriend

The aim here is to: (1) not get too heavy and serious and scare him off; (2) let him know you had a good time and want more; and (3) point out that he can stay around for as long as he likes. If he doesn't respond (because, let's face it, some boys are a little slow in the morning), try instigating some morning sex; this will stop the awkwardness and allow him to show his full appreciation of you. Avoid at all costs post-sex analysis and wedding talk.

How to tell him you'd like more

To find out if he wants to move from sex to dating, look for signals that he's interested in you as a person, not just a body with breasts. Obviously, if he finds excuses to stick around in your bed then he's interested in the sex part, but to discover the 'I like you' potential you need to get him back in his clothes, pronto. Food is a perfect option here – if he looks eager to go out for breakfast or join you in your kitchen, he definitely wants more time with you. If he says he's not hungry, keeps looking at his watch and is thumbing through the Yellow Pages for cab numbers, it's time to let him go.

He's making it clear he wants to leave

Rejection's tough but begging is the pits. The key here is dignity, with a capital 'D'. Remember, there could be a million reasons why he wants out, and the last one could be because he regrets what happened with you. Maybe he's late for work, or hitched to someone else. Even if he just wants to get away because he's embarrassed, don't get hysterical and torture yourself with what you've done wrong – just let him go.

Babe pointers

+ **Have a sense of humour** It will get you far when it comes to morning-after etiquette, especially if you feel embarrassed and awkward about what you're going to do next.
+ **Remember he feels awkward too** So don't babble, mother him or make him feel as if he's broken into your house. Be clear about what you want to happen next and he will follow your lead.
+ **Don't give him a morning-after critique** Yes, humour works, but joking about his performance or overanalysing what went on is bad news all round. Leave the analysis for your friends and, if you want him to leave, get up and start getting dressed – he'll follow your lead.
+ **Don't get scary** Especially if you like him! Being scary means asking what you'll call your kids, talking about weddings and suggesting something that veers on the wicked and wild side of sex.

How to put the oomph back into long-term sex

 Remember the time when sex was so phenomenal? When your sexual urges overtook everything else in your life? Well, the good news is that no matter how uninspired your carnal life has become, you can reclaim the excitement by simply adding a naughty risk component to your sexual adventures. Partake in some dangerous and risky loving, say the experts, and you'll reap thrill benefits similar to those of extreme sports. Do something sexually daring and you'll activate the body's 'fight or flight' response, releasing adrenalin waves into the body, boosting sexual-excitement levels and orgasm potential. Here's how to add the danger, while minimising the consequences.

Outdoor sex

High risk – OK, it's illegal, so there's the law to think about … plus it's potentially embarrassing and probably not a good way to make your family proud. However, in spite of these obvious killjoys there is much to be said in favour of outdoor orgasms. For starters, it takes a certain brazenness and speed to have sex in the wild open – meaning quickie sex will take on a whole new lease of life for both of you. Plus, the fear of being discovered can bring your arousal levels practically up to his speed enhancing the chances of a simultaneous orgasm.

Naughty pics

Medium risk – photographs, videos and home movies … this is your chance to be a Hollywood couple. However, we're not talking 'Readers' Wives' here – so choose your tools (and I mean that literally) carefully. A handy cheap camera will do, but how will you explain yourself when your film is confiscated for being obscene? Also beware new technology unless you trust your partner 100 per cent – it's just a short step from your own personal computer file to having your bits emailed around the world. A better option is a Polaroid camera (no negatives).

Act up

Role-play – as in pretending to be someone different or acting out fantasy scenarios – has a high impact but is low risk, as you're only *pretending* to have an affair/meet a strange man in a bar. Tempted to play this one for real? Well, it's worth noting that while 33 per cent of men say they'd have an affair if the chance arose, 70 per cent say it's always harmful to a relationship and over 40 per cent would never forgive being betrayed. However, while affairs happen for a variety of reasons, it is possible to incorporate the sexual thrill of the the-more-you-have-to-lose-the-better-sex-feels into your own sex life through role-play. By harnessing the elements that make sex with someone different so tempting you can bring your sex life to a higher and more satisfying level.

Babe pointers

✦ **Don't force the issue** You may be turned on by the idea of a new sexual experience, but be careful about how you introduce the issue. Be too blatant or too pushy and you'll not only turn your partner off but also leave him feeling he's not enough for you.

✦ **Start small** Think about changing how and when you have sex. Try a quickie before you go to work and/or sex on Saturday at lunchtime instead of Saturday at 10.00 p.m. (supposedly the most common time to have sex). All of these things bring back a thrill of excitement to long-term sex.

✦ **Do something different** Bored because you know all his moves? Well, he probably feels the same way. Stuck for ideas? Then rent a porn video, read a sex book or ask your friends for their naughty tips.

✦ **Change location** A change is sometimes as good as a rest, so if you can't afford to go on holiday, take the sex out of the bedroom and into another room, or even out of bed and on to the floor.

emotions

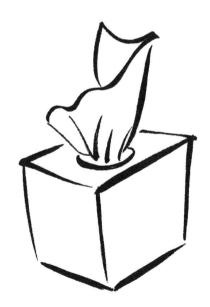

How to deal with the blues

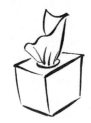

If you feel depressed, blue, under the weather and/or tired of life, you're not alone. The World Health Organisation currently estimates that depression affects 340 million people worldwide. The good news is you don't have to suffer alone. Whether your blues are short-lived or lingering, you can get help that will not only help banish the dark times but literally make you feel like a new person. Here's how.

Ask for professional help

The first step for anyone who feels depressed is to visit their doctor as soon as possible, as he or she is an essential source of information about possible treatments. While this can be a tough step to take, it's your doctor who will able to offer you a whole range of treatments and reassure you that you don't have to go through this alone. The road most people go down is either anti-depressants or counselling, or both together. If, however, you feel confused by the many different types of therapy available, bear in mind that all counselling approaches have the same goal – that you get better and feel better by bringing the stuff on the inside out to the outside.

See your blues as a learning curve

Feeling depressed isn't a sign you're failing or have failed, but a way of rethinking your strategy for life. It usually occurs once you realise your current strategy isn't working, and it's a withdrawal from society to give yourself time to think. Plenty of people go through a period of withdrawal before they emerge to reconquer their world.

Take up a physical activity

Thinking too much can be exhausting, which is where exercise can help with the blues. As exercise is tough work on your body, it literally forces you to live in the present and focus on your breathing. Just an hour a day is a good way of breaking your thoughts and getting your body into shape as well. Exercise also increases serotonin levels in the brain in much the same way that anti-depressants do. This in turn boosts your mood and helps release the body's natural painkillers – endorphins – to heighten this feelgood reaction.

Talk about how you feel ...

... to your friends and family and anyone you trust. You may think talking is overrated but you'd be amazed at how a problem shared is a problem halved. When you talk, be sure to ask for what you want, that is, do you just need to talk, or are you looking for advice? Choose a person who you know has a sensible head, not someone who will start telling you their life story halfway through your tale. Finally, talking can help you to feel less despairing, as sharing your worries often helps you to see that: (1) all is not lost; (2) you are not by yourself in this world; and (3) there is always hope.

Babe pointers

+ **Keep a diary** If you can't face talking to anyone, start writing a diary, so that you can let loose with your feelings and get negative thoughts out of your head. Think about writing it at night before you sleep (it's also a good insomnia cure) and then not reading it until morning.

+ **Pamper yourself** Also known as: treat yourself as if you were on holiday. Lie back and watch some films that make you laugh, eat lovely foods and lie in the bath.

+ **Give yourself a break** It's impossible always to be happy in life and so there will naturally be times when you feel blue and down. When this happens, don't make it worse by being hard on yourself – take time out, sit back and remind yourself these feelings will eventually pass.

+ **Give yourself a two-week deadline** If after that time you still feel depressed, seek professional help – feeling that life has no point or entertaining thoughts of self-harm is a warning signal that you need help.

How to believe in yourself

 If you think you are a fake at your job, worry that you can't be the person others think you are, feel perplexed by instructions and cry when shouted at, it's time to get a grip and start believing in yourself. Remember: it pays to be your own cheerleader (let's face it, who else will be if you won't?) for a number of reasons, including: it feels good; it makes others treat you with more respect; and it helps you to go further than you ever thought you could. Take a deep breath and learn how.

Exorcise your past

The past doesn't have to equal the future unless you let it. Lots of people overcome terrible backgrounds and slurs against their personality and mistakes, and you can, too. Whether you were bullied at school or told you were useless by a parent, teacher or ex, it's time to kick back and regain some of your lost power.

The only thing that matters is what you think of yourself, not what someone in the past thought. You may once have been useless at sport/maths/relationships, but that doesn't mean you are now. Step away from the past, live in the present and plan for the future.

Find a role model

Someone who has beaten the odds, or just generally impresses you with the way they run their life. If you can't think of anyone in your everyday life, find a hero on TV, in books – even a fictional one – who you find inspiring, and use their techniques to your advantage. For example, if it's a famous woman, what makes her so appealing? Could you grab some of this too? What makes her successful? How can you harness some of her motivation and vigour for life?

List your successes

You may feel an out-and-out failure but what are your past successes? What are you proud of? Maybe it's your nature, your friendships, the way you care about the environment or politics, or how you got out of a bad relationship and learnt from it. The list is endless, if you start seeing value in what you've already got rather than what you haven't.

Make a plan

If you want to believe in yourself, you have to start from the bottom, and to perform better you need a plan. Think about who you want to be a year from now, and write it down. List career achievements, romantic gains, body hopes, and then five things you want to do or learn in the next 12 months that are purely for fun. Your aim is to open up your life to new experiences that will teach you not only how to have more confidence in yourself but also how to value your strengths and weaknesses. So take a deep breath – and just do it!

Babe pointers

+ **Do something scary every day** This means scary, not risky. It could be: talk to a person who makes you feel shy; ask someone out; sign up for the gym; or call an old friend. The aim is to move out of your comfort zone so you can start feeling braver about life.
+ **So what if you can't do something?** It's not the end of the world if you don't like scuba diving, parachuting or plain old driving. You don't have to keep doing these things to prove you can do them. It's better to find some other interests that help boost your confidence.
+ **Don't let anxiety distract you** Worrying that others think you're weak/pathetic/useless is a waste of your time. What's important is what you think, not how others might or might not perceive you.
+ **Ignore stereotypes** So what if no girl from your background ever won an Oscar? You can be the first. Life is made up of a whole list of firsts who were always being told they couldn't do something.

How to win any argument

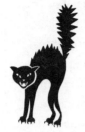

Ask anyone who's good at debating and you'll find that there's a fine art to winning an argument effectively, and contrary to popular belief it has little to do with shouting and being a smartypants. In effect, winning an argument has as much to do with your technique – body language, eye contact, tone of voice – as it does with what you say. To get your opponent to gush with apology, accept you are right and even agree with you, here's what you need to know.

It's all down to confidence

Otherwise known as: act like you're right. This is not an invitation to be smug, aggressive and/or passive-aggressive but a chance to use body language to your advantage. Look and sound like you know what you're talking about and you'll be amazed at how quickly people will crumble. Confident body language is about maintaining good posture, letting your shoulders stay down as you talk, holding in your stomach and letting your arms hang loose by your sides as you maintain eye contact. A confident tone of voice is achieved if you speak at an even pace and timbre and ensure that you don't make your sentences go up at the end (a sure sign that you are unsure of what you're saying).

Stay calm

Lose your rag and you risk losing the argument. Nothing will make the other person assume you're wrong faster than arguing too loudly and too aggressively, so think calmness at all times. If you lose your temper quickly, take regular breaths and count to ten before you say something. This gives your brain time to stop and think and work out the best thing to say. To calm someone else down, try to match your voice to theirs; if they're talking too fast, come in slightly slower just under them. Matching vocal tones has an immediate calming effect and will make the person you're talking to think you're agreeing with them.

Have a strategy

Whatever your argument, it always pays to have a strategy so you know where you're coming from and where you're going. It will help when things heat up and help when you feel you've lost your way. The four key components are: (1) know your point; (2) stick to it; (3) don't confuse the issue; and (4) know what you want. Mess up on any of the above and you risk coming away not only dissatisfied but also confused about what you're arguing about.

Don't panic

Keep things in perspective and you'll keep a firm hold on the argument. If you're seeing red over small issues, you need to work out what you're really fighting about. Is it something larger you're afraid to confront, or is it more important for you to be right than to be happy in this relationship (be it with a work colleague, partner, friend or family member)? Don't let the adrenalin of arguing throw you into a panic where becoming the winner is your only aim. If all else fails, back down gracefully – it may not feel like you've won the argument, but it will ensure you maintain your dignity!

Babe pointers

+ **Know your opponent** Some people love fighting, some hate being confronted. Work out who you're facing and plan your strategy accordingly.
+ **Know your warning triggers** We all have triggers that spiral an argument out of control. Know yours and how to combat them and you'll be able to control any discussion to your advantage.
+ **Don't shout** And while you're at it, don't name-call and make this a fight about everything. Keep to the point, be specific and speak in a calm, restrained voice, and you'll win the argument.
+ **Be gracious** Especially if you win – everyone hates a smug winner, and if you act smug, then even though you'll have won the fight you'll have lost everyone's respect.

How to stop worrying

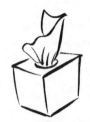

Are you the world's greatest worrier – someone who stresses about the big stuff, the small stuff and then stuff in between; a fretter whose mind plays like a broken record cataloguing a list of things that might go wrong? If you spoil every event for yourself with constant worries, and drive your friends mad with your pessimism and fear, it's time to get a grip and break the chain of worry. Here's how.

Don't always anticipate the worst

Worriers are plagued with the internal voice of doom; the voice that insists on listing every plague that could potentially fall on your head in every situation. The problem is that anticipating the worst doesn't actually protect you from the worst happening – usually because the very thing you don't think to anticipate is usually the thing that ends up knocking

you off-centre. Plus, if it doesn't happen, all you've done is waste a whole load of energy worrying about nothing.

Differentiate between good worrying and bad worrying

Good worrying is a form of problem-solving: it can help you work out where you have gone wrong or where you might go wrong in a situation. However, toxic worrying (where you worry endlessly and go round in a circle) interferes with your ability to think rationally and just makes situations worse for you. A good clue that you're going down the latter path is that you're worrying that bad things might happen when everything is going well.

Don't worry alone

Worry is damaging when it's done in isolation because that's when you're more likely to blow things out of proportion, turn small events into catastrophes and imagine the world is going to cave in on you. Talk over the problem with someone who is not a worrier so you can ground your worries in reality. For example, it's

OK to worry that a man you like may not call, but it's foolish to worry that he's going to cheat on you and break your heart before you've even gone on a date together.

Have a plan

Take action against your worries instead of letting them poison your mind. This means calling up your bank if you're getting into debt, or seeing a doctor if you're worried about a lump on your arm. Not only will taking positive action put you back in control of your life, but it will make you feel less vulnerable and, therefore, you will worry less.

Learn to let go

Some things are impossible to solve: a friend's behaviour that's always getting her into trouble; the way your mum won't do anything but watch TV; the economy taking a nose-dive – the list is endless, so learn what to stress about and what to let go of. Worry is a habit, and you can spend all your time doing it if you don't make a conscious effort to choose your worries wisely.

Babe pointers

✦ **Change your focus** Instead of thinking about what could go wrong, think about what could go right. Our mind believes what we tell it: fill it with high hopes and potentially good turns of luck, and that's what you'll start expecting.

✦ **Shout STOP!** Every time you find yourself in a worry cycle, stop instantly, take some deep breaths and immediately think of three good things that might occur. This is the way to break a chain of worry.

✦ **Don't be led by others** Worrying is contagious, so be aware of who you are listening to, and why. If you feel yourself getting nervous, anxious and fearful, work out if this is the right response to a situation, or something you're picking up from others.

✦ **Don't use worry as an excuse** If worrying has stopped you going after the man/job/promotion that you want, then you're using potential catastrophes as an excuse. Remember: nothing ventured, nothing gained.

How to feel more in control

It's worth starting this section with an essential piece of advice: being controlling and feeling in control are basically two very different things. One has more to do with fear and the other more to do with being free. How can you tell which is which? Well, if you're someone who won't do something silly just for a laugh/try something new and/or venture off your square of security, then it's likely you are relatively controlling (have your friends ever mentioned this?) and probably don't feel very in control at all. So here's how to balance the scales.

Face your anxiety

To feel more in control (and be less controlling) you have first to look at how much anxiety you have circling around in your head. While a certain amount of anxiety is normal and natural, it's important to get your fears into perspective. Whereas you can't control your surroundings, you can control your responses. Meaning instead of letting anxiety paralyse you, use your fears to push you into taking risks and looking at problems face on.

Arm yourself with information

Information is power – so if you feel insecure and out of control about a situation, grab more information before you do anything. Finding out facts will not only bring you more clarity but also help you make choices as to how you can respond. For example, if you're worried about a work presentation, first find out how many people you're presenting to. Next consider the length of the presentation and then seek out information on the best way to perform.

Don't over-commit yourself

This is a classic way to feel out of control in life. Knowing your limitations is the key to feeling in control. If you're bad with time management, don't tell people you can run three projects in two different places. If your people skills are poor, don't apply for a job that has you working with ten or more people. Turn the negatives into positives by emphasising the fact that whereas you can't run a number of projects simultaneously you're great at working independently and without support.

Make decisions

That doesn't mean all the decisions, but decisions that are good for you, even if you just make them in your head. Whereas it's tempting to be a people-pleaser and say yes to everything, if you know a group holiday is a recipe for disaster for you, opt out, or at least find a compromise, such as you have your own room. This way you can feel in control of the situation without being controlling.

Don't manage people

It's tempting to try to control situations in an underhand way by subtly managing people without their knowing. Setting up situations to your advantage isn't being in control but being manipulative. Work on managing yourself. If you know your own mind and are willing to stand by your decisions, you won't feel the need to manage others all the time.

Babe pointers

✦ **Relax** There's nothing like fatigue and tiredness to make you feel out of control and under stress. Take time out simply to do nothing. Take regular holidays and ensure you have time just to lie back and think.

✦ **Ask for help** No one expects you to do everything on your own. So if you feel out of control, ask for help in any way you can: stretch a deadline, ask for support, or simply change arrangements.

✦ **Practise good time management** There's nothing more likely to make you feel out of control than rushing from one place to the next. Don't over-commit yourself socially or fill your time with so many appointments there's literally no time to get from A to B or to enjoy it when you get there.

✦ **Smell the roses** As in: stop and look around you and enjoy what you have. One good way to feel in control is to see all the good things you have in your life and notice how you managed to get them without asserting control over others.

How to get on with your partner

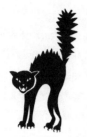

Bickering, fighting, arguing, sulking and generally annoying each other – is this a good description of how you and your partner get on? If so, it's likely you either think this is normal couple behaviour or generally assume everyone does this when they love each other. While the above is certainly a form of communication, it's probably not one worth recommending. For starters it's demoralising, leads to relationship insecurity and generally isn't a good definition of what love should be. Plus it's horrible for others to be around, and exhausting for the two of you. Want to change your ways? Here's how.

Consider the obvious
If late nights out, too much alcohol and fast food are making you feel lethargic, overtired and grumpy, you are more likely to lose your temper over something small and/or blow something meaningless out of proportion. So do yourself a favour and get healthy; it will be good not only for your body but also for your head and your love life. Eight hours sleep a night, less fast food (all that sugar causes manic highs and lows) and less booze all round.

How do you fight?
Studies show that how couples fight reflects whether or not they are made to stay together. If you're a 'bring-everything-to-the-party' kind of girl, it's likely a small argument about what TV show to watch becomes a diatribe about every annoying thing your partner does. If so, you're killing your relationship. Deal with the point in hand and work on the rest when you're both calmer. At the same time, learn to defuse harsh words with humour and take part of the blame in situations (even if you don't feel you are to blame), as this is the healthy compromise for the bigger picture.

Stop the bickering
Bickering is slow poison but it's weirdly addictive to do. If you find yourself

nagging, griping or being attacked in this way it's worth noting that a lot of bickering comes from what's known as the 'shadow syndrome'. This is when you (or your partner) see the parts you don't like in yourself in the person you love and try to change them. Like many habits, it can be broken by your taking a step back and consciously seeing what you're doing to your partner and your relationship.

Don't stop kissing each other

Studies show that couples who kiss stay together longer and are happier. Don't forget to show the small stuff even when you're angry. A kiss, a nice gesture, even 'I love you even though you make me crazy' can defuse a situation and help remind you of why you're together.

Don't become your parents

It sounds scary but this is what happens to a lot of couples. We take on our parents' personae in relationships because it's the one relationship we know best. If your parents had good getting-on tactics, that's great, but sadly most of us tend to pick up the bad stuff. A good clue is if you think you're becoming your mother, you probably are!

Babe pointers

+ **Treat him like your best friend** If you wouldn't yell at her for something, don't yell at him. Likewise, don't take your bad day out on him, or if you do, at least apologise for it (it goes a lot further than you think).
+ **Set up boundaries with each other** If you continually fight about the same issue, set up mutual boundaries for what's acceptable to fight about and what isn't. The idea here is that it's not about getting your own way but about which compromises you can live with.
+ **Work out your peace ratio** If you're fighting more than you're loving, you probably have bigger problems than you want to admit. Step back and reassess what's going on. Does this relationship really have a future?
+ **Don't blame your hormones** So you're emotional and grumpy around your period – it's not his fault; don't use it as an excuse to let rip. Yes, your hormones are raging, but you can control them.

How to deal with your anger

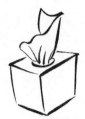

There are many types of anger: the rational you-did-this-to-me-and-now-I-am-angry-with-you kind of anger; the spoilt, petulant you-won't-do-this-for-me-and-so-I-am-mad variety; and, of course, the loud, frightening I-have-no-control-over-my-anger-and-it's-out-of-proportion-to-what's-happened kind of fury. In between there are also many other rages and temper tantrums all fuelled in part by the idea of an intolerable injustice. If you're someone who regularly runs through the whole spectrum of anger shades, then it's probably time to do some anger management.

Work out what kind of anger queen you are

Overall, anger types are divided into exploders (those who throw massive fits of rage) and imploders (those who bottle up their anger until they go nuclear with rage). If you're the former it's likely you already know you have a problem with your anger, but if you're in the latter category it's likely you don't (or won't admit it). Knowing how your anger impacts on others and your scare rating can help you to determine the level of help you need: professional, if you're scaring people and loved ones; self-control, if you need to know how to rein it in.

Keep your anger in proportion to the event

Being angry happens when you feel that somehow your needs aren't being met, so you feel hurt and/or taken for granted or walked over, and then react by getting mad. Anger's not a bad thing if it's in proportion to what's happened. Someone's rude to you – by all means get angry. Someone pushes past you by accident and apologises – getting angry is not the right response.

Defuse your short fuse

If you can't defuse your anger here's how to calm yourself down. First, count up to ten before you do anything, breathing deeply. This stops your body going into the fight/flight stress scenario that releases adrenalin into your body. Then remove yourself from the situation physically. If you're still steaming with anger, do something physical: go for a run or walk, and think about what's frustrating you and causing your anger to flare up on such a constant basis.

Talk about it

Sit down with someone and talk about how you feel and why. Consider if you simply have too high expectations of others, or if small events are triggering past events that you haven't dealt with. Or is it that you're simply under stress and suffering from fatigue, and an unhealthy lifestyle is giving you a short fuse? When you have some answers, consider how you can combat these by changing your life.

Babe pointers

✦ **Look at who you're hurting** Apart from making loved ones feel uncomfortable and even wary of you, getting angry all the time is bad for your own health. It raises your blood pressure and floods your body with the stress hormone cortisol, which is why you may feel emotionally drained after losing it.

✦ **If you're angry, say it** As in: simply and calmly say, 'I'm angry with you,' and then tell them why and what will make it better (an apology, a refund, or a change in behaviour).

✦ **Some people are horrible** The truth is some people are just nasty and plain rude. If you're unfortunate enough to come across someone like this, no amount of raging will help. Instead, remind yourself that they haven't done it to annoy you, but because they are an idiot.

✦ **Don't expect perfection** Life's unfair and sometimes, no matter what, it's annoying. Don't let anger spoil your enjoyment of life. Know how to calm down when you feel anger rising.

How to forgive someone

 So your life has more twists and turns than a guest on Jerry Springer's show; your best friend stole your boyfriend; an ex treated you cruelly and then ditched you on Valentine's Day; your boss stole your ideas and got promoted for them? You're 100 per cent right to feel annoyed, angry and downright mad. However, take a time check: how long have you been holding your grudge? Are you counting off weeks, months or even years? If the timeline seems long, it's time to stop the festering, and forgive. Here's how.

Look at how far you've come

Holding a grudge and being angry with someone can go on for so long that you can eventually just get used to the feeling and forget that it's not normal and healthy to live like this. If you can't or won't forgive someone for hurting you/ruining your life, start by looking at your life right here, right now. Are you happy? Are you fulfilled? Do you still feel like the same person they hurt? It's likely you don't, so why take the past with you into your new future?

What did you learn?

As horrible as it is to have someone hurt you, the learning curve can be good for you. Ask yourself what positive things you've learnt from the event. Have you learnt who your true friends are? Who to appreciate? Who you should trust and care about in the future? What your strengths are? It's likely you've learnt all this and more.

Change your focus

Being angry takes up a lot of energy and emotion, and often too big a space in your life. If you're sick of feeling mad, then all you have to do is change your focus and think forwards not backwards. Consider where you're going next, and with whom, and leave your old baggage where it belongs – in the past.

Think of forgiveness as a positive act

Too often people won't forgive because they assume it means letting someone off the hook for their behaviour. The way to rationalise this is to see that it lets *you* off the hook. Forgiving someone enables you to: (1) heal, so the past doesn't always feel like a knife piercing your heart; and (2) move on from the event. The other person has their own demons and guilt to exorcise, so your forgiveness will have more of an effect on your own life than on theirs.

Say it loud

Emotions hold power when they are not expressed, which is why it pays to air them. If you've been telling everyone how angry you've been for ages, then tell them loud and clear when you're over it and have moved on. Celebrate, in fact, have a party: call up all your friends and enjoy feeling the weight of that heavy grudge finally lifting from your shoulders.

Babe pointers

+ **You don't have to forgive and forget** This is rubbish. Forgive and move on, but forgive and forget that X lied, cheated and broke your heart – unlikely. In any case you shouldn't forget; this should act as a warning alarm in case you meet someone else who rings the same bell.

+ **Get closure** Write a letter, make a phone call, send a text – the person who hurt you may not care if you forgive them or not, but if it makes you feel closure, go for it.

+ **Don't beat yourself up** The weird thing about forgiving is once you've done it you'll wonder why you didn't do it earlier. That's fine, because everyone has that reaction. However, avoid the 'I've wasted so much time' scenario; that's a path just not worth going down.

+ **Forgive, and mean it** As in: don't let it rear its ugly head the next time you feel down, have PMS, fear the worst in a new relationship, or bump into the person you've forgiven. Over means over!

How to curb your jealousy

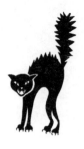

Do you regularly turn into the green-eyed monster? Does jealousy tinge all your relationships and have you hating yourself? If so, you're not alone. Everyone feels jealous and envious sometimes. However, if it's eating away at your life and relationships here's how to get control of that tricky emotion.

Jealousy is about wanting something

The feelings of jealousy arise out of our unfulfilled desires: when we want something but secretly believe we cannot have it, so we either tend to pretend that we don't want it or deny we ever wanted it, as a way of avoiding disappointment. Unfortunately, as soon as someone else comes along with that very thing, jealousy rises to the surface and we feel betrayed, hurt and left out.

Don't feel that you can't have it, too

The trick with feeling jealous is to remind yourself that someone hasn't stolen your chance of success or love or happiness; if anything, if they have it then the chances are that one day you will too. The good thing about jealousy is that it helps us to see what we really want in life. If the life of a loved-up friend makes you feel jealous, then it's likely that you also want to be loved in that way. If a sibling's job success turns us green, it's a sign that we want more job success in life. Act on the bottom line, not the overwhelming emotion.

Don't feed your jealousy

The real problem with feeling jealous is that the one person it hurts the most is you. The more you allow it to take root, the more agonising it becomes. If you keep telling yourself someone has what you want, eventually you'll feel cheated to the degree that you'll push away the very thing you want. Instead of pretending you're not feeling this way, open up and say it out loud. Apart from being a huge release, you can then at least talk about what's getting you down.

Relationship jealousy is insecurity

So don't dress it up as something else. Feeling your partner's head will be turned by the first pretty woman who comes along shows two things about you: (1) you don't believe you're good enough for him so he's bound to stray; and (2) you think so much of him, he could have anyone. The result of this kind of jealousy is suspicion, fear, anxiety and eventually relationship breakdown, as your partner gets sick of constantly reassuring you. To combat all of this you need to boost your self-esteem (*see* Life) so you feel worthy and secure of your partner and the value of your relationship.

Babe pointers

+ **Be honest** At least with yourself, because the one thing about jealousy is eventually you'll give yourself away and no one wants to be around someone who lets their jealous feelings overtake them.

+ **Don't ask for sympathy** While everyone knows what it's like to be jealous, asking a friend for sympathy because something nice has happened to her is ridiculous. It is possible to be happy for someone and jealous at the same time, so if you're going to say something, say that you're happy and then change the subject.

+ **Don't let jealousy overwhelm you** It will make you ugly. If you feel entitled to feel jealous about your best friend, eventually you'll feel jealous about a work friend, and then a sibling's life, and so on and so on … Stop the rot.

+ **Take action** It will make you feel more in control than sitting around crying about your lack of luck. If you can't learn from someone else's behaviour, make your own plan. And above all remind yourself that you're young, healthy and smart – so why are you coveting someone else's life?

How to get over things

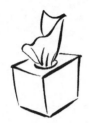

Dumped, ditched, given the old heave-ho by a friend and/or passed over at work – call it what you may, getting over disappointment is a tough old business. You want to be dignified about it, but the reality is: inside you're ready to fall apart. It's called grief, and whether you're suffering from heartbreak, a big friendship let-down or a work setback, it feels like the end of the world. Much of this has to do with our dashed expectations and feeling a door has slammed on our future which can hit very hard. Grief is a process that you simply can't get over overnight. Here's how to do it in all its various stages.

As soon as it happens

Initially, you can't breathe, never mind stand, or think. You may feel dizzy, nauseous and perhaps even a little faint. Your body's cold and clammy, and although you're not dying (even if you wish you were) you're experiencing what's known as shock. Never underestimate the physical and emotional effects of shock; help yourself by first allowing yourself to feel what's happening: scream, shout, rage – do what you need to do to get it all out.

Then lean on people and wallow in your misery for a day or two. This is what family and good friends are for – and it's your right to feel hurt, miserable and downright unhappy.

A week down the line

You should be out of shock by now, although you're probably still wading through crumpled tissues, wondering how and why it all went wrong and still hoping it was all a horrible mistake – this is known as denial. Part of the reason you feel so physically blue is because right now your levels of serotonin and dopamine – the body's feelgood chemicals – are low. The adrenal glands, which control functions that enable the body to adapt to stress, are also not working properly, which means your body is in a highly stressed state. As a result, you'll notice your eating and sleeping habits going haywire and feel high levels of anxiety and tension. Help yourself by eating chocolate and healthy foods, such as vegetables and lean meat, as these contain a chemical that will increase insulin levels in the body that will convert to serotonin in the brain, helping you to feel happier.

A month on

It's likely that depression and anger have set in, but this is the final part of getting over something. Depression occurs because you've now let go of hope, and anger kicks in because it's the only way you can now stay connected to whatever you're grieving over. The good news is that finally letting go of those Soprano-style revenge fantasies means finally moving on. And moving on is where your thoughts should be. Concentrate on working out what went wrong and how you can turn it around next time. If it's something beyond your control, then think about accepting what has happened and then make a new plan. You know what they say: as one door closes, another one opens...

Babe pointers

✦ **Find ways to relax** The brain needs time to come to terms with everything that has happened, and it can't do this if it's not in a relaxed state. Start with taking a half-hour walk somewhere calming once a day. Book a holiday, take time out for yourself, and have some massages and beauty treatments to pamper yourself.

✦ **Look after yourself** Resolve to avoid takeaways and too much alcohol. Get some regular exercise and don't deprive yourself of sleep, or drink yourself to sleep. Excesses of any kind won't help when you're trying to get over something.

✦ **Don't wallow** By the six-week mark you should be able to look back and see how far you've come. If you haven't moved at all, you're wallowing and need to look forwards and not backwards.

✦ **Break the chain** Also known as: let go of what could have been. Until you do this you'll never be able to get over anything.

friendships

How to listen and be listened to

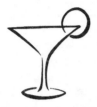 Thinking you are a good listener is akin to thinking you have style. Everyone thinks they excel at it, but not everyone can. The fact is that some people are just useless at listening but, ironically, feel they are 'excellent' listeners. Either they get easily distracted or they are simply not used to focusing for long periods and so just lose the connection. The real culprits here, of course, are those people who tune out after the second sentence, and usually long before you've got to the point, causing you to say accusingly, 'You're not listening, are you?' while they deny it with their very last breath. Sick of missing the point and/or not being heard? Here's how to fine-tune those listening skills.

Keep to the point

If you want people to listen, it's a question of less detail and more fact. Keep your conversations short and sharp in order to get your point across. A person does not need to know what you had for breakfast if you're telling them how you got stuck in traffic on the way to work. Always start with your key point and work backwards to grab their attention and hold it.

Listen as much as you talk

You probably think you do, but you probably don't. If you don't believe me, check your watch and time how long you can hold off before butting back into a conversation. If you really do say hardly anything then it's time to be assertive with your listening skills. Interrupt, ask people to stick to the point and, if you still lose track, repeat the last thing they say as it will make them remember what they were saying.

Practise attentive listening

Simply just listen to someone speak and, when you feel yourself drifting, consciously pull yourself back into the moment by either breathing deeply, or pinching yourself. The aim here is to nod, make sounds and empathise without actually saying anything. This is an essential listening skill because, often, friends in need want to talk and are not asking for a life-saving plan of action from you.

Don't bring the conversation back round to yourself

This is where most people go wrong when listening. Repeat: you do not have to say anything remotely helpful. You do not have to talk about yourself, you do not have to jump in when the other person stops for breath, and you do not have to yawn because you're bored. Finally, if the person has been talking for hours and you really have listened and heard nothing of interest, you do have the right simply to walk away.

Babe pointers

✦ **Get rid of blabbers** These are people who talk and talk and talk at you. They are the people who are not really interested in you, but just want to use you as a sounding board.

✦ **If someone's not listening to you, tell them** Obvious, but hardly ever acted on. Feel misunderstood, not listened to? Don't sit there sulking and wishing things were different, speak up and ask to be heard.

✦ **Tell others what you need** Often when we're asking to be listened to, people hear that we need advice or help. This is because it's often difficult to hear someone in trouble and not say something. If you just want five minutes during which to complain, with no 'helpful' tips, say so.

✦ **Consider how good a listener you are** You may think you never get a word in but, hand on heart, are you really good at listening? Do you really hear what others say or are you simply waiting to say your piece the whole time? It may be time to start practising what you preach.

How to accept a compliment

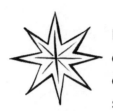

Being able to accept a compliment is the cornerstone to good self-esteem. If you readily bat away the good comments thrown your way because you think people are just being 'nice' and only trust the nasty things people say, it's time to learn how to be gracious. Compliments are essentially the way other people let you know that they think a lot of you. When you throw one back what you're saying to them is: (1) I don't trust your motives; (2) I don't think that highly of myself; and (3) I think you're lying to me. Here's how to change your perspective.

Find the correct response

Most people don't like compliments because they don't know what to say when they get one. They worry that they'll look bigheaded if they accept, and so they choose instead to throw it away. The answer, therefore, is simply to say 'Thank you' and smile. You don't have to give a compliment back, you don't have to explain why you agree, and you certainly don't then have to put yourself down to show them you're not egotistic. Also, bear in mind that to do anything besides say 'Thanks' is to make the other person feel uncomfortable, and why would you want to do that, when they've just said something nice to you?

Give out compliments

People who are good at accepting compliments tend also to give out a lot of compliments. This is because they have the self-confidence and self-esteem to realise that saying something nice makes the people they like feel good. The key is: if you think/feel something you should say it, because what's the point in just thinking it? If you can't bring yourself to compliment others, then you need to look at what's holding you back.

Look at the compliments you can't take

As these will be in the area where you're most likely to lack confidence. If you can't take someone's telling you that you look well without thinking they mean 'You're fat', or their saying that you look good without thinking they mean 'for an ugly person', then you need to boost your self-esteem (*see* You). Being able to acknowledge that you are attractive/smart/funny means you can accept all those things and more. This has nothing to do with being bigheaded, but lots to do with the fact that you are genuinely a confident person.

Trust your friends and family

There is an idea that your friends and family don't tell you the truth, and so any nice compliments tend not to count. The reality is: if anyone is going to tell you the truth it's your family and friends, so start to believe what they say! If in doubt, think about how you respond to them when they're feeling low and are in need of a confidence boost. Do you lie to them or simply tell them something nice that you truly feel?

Babe pointers

✦ **Compliment yourself** Being nice to yourself when you are looking in the mirror or have done something good is a great way to learn to live with compliments. If it sounds ridiculous it's likely you've never said anything nice to yourself, so try it now.

✦ **Have a compliment quota** Say three nice things a day to people in your life. Don't think too hard, just compliment them on the everyday and mundane.

✦ **Watch how others take compliments** It will give you tips on how to be gracious, especially if you have a hard time saying 'Thanks' to your compliments. Notice how people don't focus on the compliment but still take time to take pleasure from it.

✦ **Remember the good things people say** We're all very good at hoarding the bad comments and ignoring the good. De-clutter your brain of those bad thoughts of what someone once said to you in the playground, and start collecting the good ones.

How to widen your circle of friends

 In need of new friends because of a change in your life circumstances? Sick of the people you've known for years, or just desperate to meet and interact with new and interesting people? If so, the world is your oyster. We all assume that no one's trying to meet and make new friends simply because no one ever admits it, but the truth is most people are yearning to branch out and meet new people to help open up their world.

Of course, gone are the days when you could just walk up to someone in the school playground and ask them to be your best friend, or assume they would be because you invited them to your birthday party. These days, making new friends takes effort, and often a character reference, but it can be done. Here's how.

Act like a single person

Meaning look for friends the way you'd look for a new boyfriend. Think of all the places you go to regularly – is there anyone there who catches your eye, smiles and/or looks like the kind of person you'd want to be friends with? If so, initiate conversation with them and see if there's any mileage in the relationship. Next, accept all invitations to parties – as these are the ideal places to click with someone new. Better still, take a look at your friends' friends and see if there's anyone there that you'd like to strike up a new friendship with.

Look under every stone

Think about all the friends you have right now and how you got to know them. It's likely you didn't meet them all through school and work, but also in some pretty weird places. The key to making friends is to be open to new people wherever you are: on the bus, in a café, drinking in a pub and even in a queue.

Consider why you want new friends, and look accordingly

Knowing why you want new mates can help you to work out where to look for them. Looking for a group of single friends to go out on the pull with? Then ask your coupled friends if they know anyone. Better still, have a potluck dinner party. This is where every friend has to bring along another friend in order to help everyone meet someone new.

Work at it

Finally, bear in mind that new friendships take work and effort. Meaning you may have to spend a few weeks doing the inviting out, and maybe even pursuing someone. Don't be shy about doing this if you know that you and the person you have in mind work well together. It's flattering, and most people will jump at the chance to get to know you better.

Babe pointers

+ **De-clutter your old friendships**
Sometimes, instead of getting lots of new friends, it pays to shake up your old ones. Are your friendships stuck in a rut? Are you bored by what you all do together? If so, don't kick them to one side but think about ways you can change these friendships for the better.

+ **Try something new** Can't find a new friend anywhere? Then think about the old classics: join an evening class (language classes are the most friendly), a running group, a book group and/or a salsa class. If none of those takes your fancy, consider one of the many dinner-party clubs, which regularly arrange social events.

+ **Consider friends of different ages** You're no longer at school choosing your mates based on age and which class you're in, so think younger and older – you could well end up with the kind of friendship you're really looking for.

+ **Ask what makes you a great friend** The answer to this will help you to determine not only where you'll find friends and why, but also what your friendship quota is, that is, what your value is as a friend.

How to make a new friend

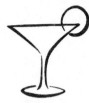 In life it pays to know how to get someone to be your friend – not just on friendship grounds but also in general, because it's the key to social and work success. Luckily it's not down to looks and intellectual intelligence but something known as 'emotional intelligence'. Also known as: how well you read someone and act on those signals. If you have no idea what I am talking about, it's likely you are the person who blunders in when others know to hold back. So if you're sick of putting your foot in it and tired of having others misread you, here's how to make a social impact.

Read body language

As 55 per cent of the signals we send out and receive are through body language, it pays to know how to read someone. Clues that they're interested in talking to you include: leaning towards you when you talk; making eye contact; and general assertive behaviour as you speak. Signs they aren't interested include: looking over your shoulder as you speak; moving away from you as you get closer; and giving you monosyllabic answers. If the latter's what you're getting, move on; this person's not worth getting to know. Find someone more receptive and open to you.

Build trust

If you get positive feedback, start building a bond between you by emphasising the common ground you share. This makes a person feel comfortable because it makes them feel as if their beliefs are being affirmed. Obviously, don't overdo it because then they'll feel as if you aren't being authentic and will back off. Finally, even if you have hundreds of interests in common, always be sure to listen as much as you speak.

Don't be pushy

In the same way that you wouldn't be pushy with a prospective boyfriend, don't be pushy with a new friend. Give them your number, swap email addresses and suggest you do something together and then sit back and wait. Sending them 23 texts in a day and/or calling them every day is overkill. Likewise, not returning someone's calls, using them as a stopgap when you're bored, or generally ditching them at the last minute won't cement your friendship in any way whatsoever.

Three strikes

Finally, work on the 'three strikes and you're out' principle. Call them, ask them out and wait. If they cancel, don't take it personally, just try again and see what their return value is. If after three attempts they've either made countless excuses and/or wriggled out of things, work out if you still want to be friends with them. If not, back off – and try again with someone else.

Don't spill all your dirty laundry

When you make a connection it can be tempting to lay your life story at someone's feet – don't! Not only is it off-putting but also it sends out the signal that you're intense and hard work. Have some laughs first and save the tougher stuff for later.

Babe pointers

✦ **Offer a wide range of options** Not everyone is comfortable coming to a party or club; some people prefer one-to-one encounters, others small gatherings. To discover what people like best, offer a range of get-together options and see what grabs them.

✦ **Look for friends with common interests** It sounds obvious, but most people don't look under their noses for friends. If you want a friendship to last it has to be built on more than two things.

✦ **Don't be afraid to say no to someone** Likewise, you don't have to be friends with everyone who offers you an outstretched palm. Choose your friends wisely, not because you feel bad about saying no.

✦ **Keep your distance** As tempting as it is to see someone all the time when you first meet, distance does actually make a friendship closer. Take your time, there's no rush, don't let the friendship burn out before it's even had a chance to work.

How to deal with a difficult friend

Friends can be difficult for all kinds of reasons. Some are made that way, while others have problems that start to affect all of their relationships. Then there are those who are going through a stressful period and/or simply taking out their anger/temper/emotions on you. Whatever their problem, if it's become your problem too, it's time to act. Here's how.

Stand up for yourself

It should be relatively simple: a friend is rude/difficult/annoying, you say so, they apologise and everything's rosy again. Unfortunately, relationships and friendships are trickier than that, which is why most of us don't confront the issue until it's too late. If you want to save a friendship and your sanity, it always pays to stand up to a friend who's being difficult. Take a deep breath and just tell them to stop doing what they're doing.

Don't be too understanding

Also known as: you are not their therapist, so you don't have to be 100 per cent understanding of their moods. OK, so you understand that your single best friend is acting up because you've got a new boyfriend and that's something she wants, but walking on eggshells with her is not the answer. The trick is to empathise with her situation (that is to try to understand what's behind her behaviour), without letting her treat you like a punch-bag for it.

Ask her what's wrong

This is the quickest way to defuse a friend's difficult behaviour, as long as you phrase it correctly. Saying 'What the hell's wrong with you then?' tends to get a negative answer, whereas 'This is so unlike you – what's up?' will get you a more positive response that you may even be able to help with. If she shuts down or refuses to let you know, then at least you've let her know that: (1) you've noticed; and (2) you've tried to help.

Tell her how she is making you feel

If none of the above helps, then simply tell her how her behaviour is making you feel. This will let your friend know that she's putting your friendship at risk and also that she's hurt you. Of course, a very difficult friend will shrug this off and/or turn it on you. If this happens, you have two choices – put some space between you or enforce some tough love on her.

Come up with workable solutions

When confronting a difficult person, the ideal way to voice it is to have solutions on hand alongside your complaints. Unsure of what might help? Then think about what would make her friendship right for you. Less talk about her/more talk about you? Fewer Bridget Jones-style conversations/more going out? Less bullying/more friendship? Only you can say!

Babe pointers

✦ **Don't wait too long to act** Or else your rage will explode and suddenly one difficult incident will become a whole list of difficult incidents that neither of you will be able to come back from.

✦ **Make sure it isn't you** This is a hard one, but sometimes friends become difficult in response to something we do to them. Have an honest look at yourself to see if you have triggered any kind of behaviour (if in doubt ask them).

✦ **Have some tolerance** OK, so she's annoying/ridiculous and downright silly but then you're not perfect either, so have some tolerance for your friends. They don't have to be replicas of you or even think the same way.

✦ **Don't be too quick to dump them** Unlike many other relationships, good friendships can last a lifetime. So, before you erase a friend from your address book, make sure that you have at least tried every avenue there is to repair the problem.

How to deal with me-me-me friends

 Me-me-me friends are the friends who constantly talk about their problems/ stresses/illnesses and love lives. They are the friends who never let you get a word in, not because they're not interested but because they simply assume you have everything sussed and so don't need to be listened to the way they do. Sadly, most are completely unaware of how needy they are and often wrongly assume they couldn't possibly be boring you. Sadly, if you're the person having to listen, the tedium is probably killing you. Here's how to cope if you've got advice fatigue.

Don't get sucked into the drama

It's a fact of life that some people are just plain complainers and love being in a constant state of hysteria and panic. Apart from giving them the Oscar for best performance in a drama – leave them to it. Letting them draw you into a supporting role not only is exhausting but also makes *your* life about *theirs*.

Have a time limit for listening

So they are heartbroken (again), crying on your shoulder (again) and making all the same old mistakes (again), but this doesn't mean you have to give them hours of your time. Talking helps, but endless talking doesn't help anyone. For your sake and theirs, set time limits for their 'chats' by pointing out that going over the same event countless times only makes them relive the pain, not remove it.

Don't be their therapist

Tempting as it is to want to help them, don't turn into a surrogate therapist. First, be aware that they may not want to sort out their problems, something that's very common among people who like to talk. The fact is that if their problems are that serious, you need to send them to a real therapist, not tell them what to do. If they aren't that serious, then they have no right to burden you all the time. Again, set limits: half an hour of unburdening and then move on to more interesting topics (this counts for phone conversations, too).

Remind them that you haven't had fun together for ages

And remind them that your friendship has to be about more than constant angst. If you become their 'agony aunt', they'll never see you as the friend they can also have fun with, and so your friendship will never move beyond the boundaries of their woes. Change the goal posts by avoiding close intimate situations with them and going out in groups. Better still, hold back on the advice. If they don't get a response from you, they won't keep talking.

Be honest

This is essentially what friendship is about, so if you can't be honest and tell them how they are making you feel, what are you getting out of this friendship? When being honest, also be kind. Someone having a tough time needs tough love but needs it in a soft way.

Babe pointers

✦ **Don't overload yourself with needy friends** If you find you do, you need to look at how you might be encouraging it. Is having lots of needy friends a way to avoid talking about yourself and your own problems? Do you yearn to be needed? Only you can say.

✦ **Talk about other things** As in: move the conversation away from the personal by talking about external things such as films, books and TV, to encourage a wider scope of interests between you.

✦ **Have the same number of sane friends** For your own sanity – because emotional overload is contagious, and you run the risk of becoming your worst nightmare.

✦ **Laugh about it** OK, she thinks she's living in a soap opera, acts like she has the life of a diva and expects you to pick up the pieces when she falls apart. It's stressful but it can also be funny – get her to laugh at herself and you're halfway to getting her to lighten up.

How to make your friends like each other

It's a cruel twist of fate that sometimes the two people you like the most in the whole world will not only loathe each other, but also be quick to make that fact clear to you. Save stranding them on a desert island together, there are a few ways to get them hooked up and friendly. So if birthday gatherings are a nightmare owing to friends' falling out with each other, here's how to get them to behave.

Reassure them that you're still friends

Unless there has been a major upset, friends who don't get on tend to stay at polar opposites owing to territorial issues – the territory being you. This is because not only are most people afraid that they will lose their friends, but when they have to meet another 'good' friend, it just makes them realise how dispensable they really are. To quash this insecurity, which can cause heaps of problems, your job is to reassure all that there's enough space in your heart for everyone, and enough time in your week for all.

Emphasise the common ground

To get friends to get on, you have to let them know what they have in common besides you, which means taking yourself out of the equation when you're all together. Don't say, 'X and I went to this art exhibition that you would have loved,' say, 'X is really into that artist you like,' and so on, and then leave them to it. Common ground can be literally anything, so just drop in a few links and then walk away and leave them to it.

Don't fuel the competition

Sometimes we can revel in the way our friends don't get on simply because we're secretly pleased they still like us best. If this is the case, either don't introduce them to each other or leave the

124

playground behind and let them be friends. This means no behind-the-scenes stirring and no gossiping about what went on without you.

Ask them both for their help in a crisis

Better still, ask them to work together for your sake. A crisis is more likely to get people to behave and try with each other; plus, as you've made yourself the common ground, they both have a focal point to remind them of their link to you. If that doesn't work, it's time to get them to focus on the bigger picture, that is, getting on for *your* sake. After all there's nothing wrong with asking for a quiet life.

Don't sweat it if they don't like each other

Sometimes you can try every trick in the book and still nothing will help two people to become friends. If that's the case, don't play the middleman. Leave problems between them, and don't avoid inviting them places together. Everyone is big enough and old enough to cope with someone they don't like. It only becomes a problem if you let it and walk on tiptoes. Remember: you don't like everyone and they don't have to either.

Babe pointers

+ **Get rid of your top ten** People act out (or, rather, act badly) when they feel their position is threatened. Are you valuing all your friends equally or letting them know there's a hierarchy and they're not scoring very high? If so, it's time to let go of your playground mentality.

+ **Let your friends get to know each other** For your sake as well as theirs. After all, there's nothing worse than hearing about how brilliant someone is all the time and yet never being introduced to them.

+ **Value your friends for different things** OK, we all have our favourites, but for the sake of all your friends, it's important to value them all for what they bring to your life. Let them know and they'll be less worried when you tell them about other friends.

+ **Be a good friend yourself** Meaning when you don't like someone else's friends, treat them as if they were their family. You don't have to like them, but you do have to be nice and polite to them.

How to be a good friend

 Being a good friend is like having good taste: everyone thinks they've got it sussed until someone points out that they haven't. Contrary to popular belief it takes more than sticking around and having a laugh to be a good friend. If you're constantly losing friends, finding your calls go unanswered and feeling surprised when a friend accuses you of being a good-time pal, here's how to change your ways.

Make time for them

So you're there for the important events – birthdays, drink-ups and Christmas – but what about the times when your friends are low and need a shoulder to cry on? Too busy with your own life to pop round for ten minutes? If so, it's worth considering that the phrase 'make time for your friends' means make time for the good times and the bad. While you don't have to be on call 24/7, a good friend will drop everything in a crisis, and most things for a good time. Make your friends always feel as if they are being slotted into your busy schedule and all that will happen is they'll drift away.

Don't gossip about them

Obvious, but horribly tempting when you have a juicy bit of news. The thing to consider is: whose news is it really? Better still, how would you feel if the tables were turned? To stop people gossiping about you, don't gossip about them. If you hear the words, 'Don't tell anyone, but …' coming out of your mouth, stop right there – you're about to betray a confidence and you know it!

Don't be the moan queen

Familiarity doesn't breed contempt, it breeds bad habits, and one of the most common is falling into a moan rut. While your friends want to be with you through thick and thin, constant whingeing and pessimism are tough to be around (and boring as hell). Censor yourself so you're not the person who's always bringing in an element of doubt and doom. It's no fun for you and it's certainly no fun for your friends.

Avoid bitching behind their backs

Remind yourself that your friends are a reflection of your life, so if you don't like them and feel the need to bitch and gripe about them constantly, you need to ask yourself why you're friends. Of course, everyone deserves a grumble or two, but make sure the good times outweigh the bad, otherwise get the heck out of there.

Do nice things for no reason

Send a card, buy a stupid gift, buy them a latte, cut out a relevant clipping from a newspaper and send it to them – all these small things and more are what makes people realise they are special to you. You don't have to have a lot of money, make grand gestures or mix your blood together to show that you're friends; all you have to do is show some appreciation, and take the time to show them that they mean something to you.

Babe pointers

+ **Watch how others respond to each other** If you're stuck for how to be a good friend, then watch how your friends interact with each other and look for the small things that help bond a friendship and make it stronger.
+ **Admit you're wrong when you're wrong** This goes a long way to showing you're a good friend, simply because it means you're honest enough to put your friendship before your ego.
+ **Compromise** To make a friendship work, treat it the way you would treat a love affair and choose your battles wisely. Otherwise known as: compromise for the sake of your friendship and your friends.
+ **Let them love you** It sounds weird, but always being the person who lavishes on the love and support is great, but it's no fun for the other person if you don't let them reciprocate. Let them be a good friend to you too and you'll both live happily ever after.

How to keep your friendships going strong

You've always been there for her and vice versa – at the times when things were good, and the times when things were bad. Now suddenly something's blocking your friendship path and your relationship's under strain. You hate her boyfriend, she ignores your successes, and you think she's mad to want to be a stay-at-home mum. Here's how to keep your bond strong when life starts to get in the way.

Remind yourself that things change

Friendships evolve and change all the time in order to survive. So rather than focus on what you've lost over the years, think about what you've gained from your joint life experiences. Being single, being married and being apart – none of these things should herald the end of a friendship or cause more than a tremor of awkwardness between you if you're both looking at the long-term goals of your friendship.

Get rid of the competitive element

Differing life choices can bring an unwelcome competitive edge to your friendship, especially if one of you is on the road to marriage and babies, while the other is still single and/or more career-orientated.

It's important to remember that you don't have to reflect the same life choices to stay friends. To maintain and enhance your friendship, be honest about your differences and uncomfortable feelings about love and work.

Make time for each other

The key to avoiding a friendship breakdown over more material differences is to make time for each other and emphasise what is still similar between you, that is, what hasn't changed over the years. Studies show that the best predictor for longevity in a friendship is shared values, not shared paths.

Don't retreat into more comfortable friendships

It's easy as you get older to stick to friendships where your interests mix and match, and ignore your old relationships that don't tend to fit any more. What's important to remember is that you can have both quite successfully if you don't alienate one from the other. To do this, make the time you have together about your friendship, not about your new life.

Talk about your lives

Reciprocal disclosure is the real secret to strong friendships. Trading intimacies, secrets and fears as well as the good times is what makes a friendship grow. Hide your inner feelings or lay them all in her lap and refuse to listen to her and your friendship will founder and disappear. Finally, build new memories together instead of relying on old ones. If all you do is talk about the past, that's where your friendship will live. Make it present-orientated and you'll give yourselves a direction to head into.

Babe pointers

+ **Introduce each other to your new lives** As tempting as it is to keep your life in segments, it pays dividends to amalgamate your friends into your life as it evolves. Make them as much a part of your successes and failures and you'll have them for life.
+ **Make an effort with each other** It's easy to let time ruin your friendships, which is why you need to keep in touch, no matter what happens. It doesn't always have to be a girlie night out, but a small text, a quick email or even a postcard is all that's needed to keep most friendships alive.
+ **Stop arguing** Bickering can destroy a relationship, which is why the secret is to not live in each other's pockets all the time.
+ **Laugh at yourself** That's what friendships are all about. The friendships that last and last are the ones where you're more than happy to laugh at what an idiot you've been. So if you've put your foot in it or made a huge blunder, call up your friend and tell her now!

129

How to survive the in-laws

There are plenty of sticky issues to face when you finally have to meet your loved one's family. Overbearing, controlling mothers and silent fathers, not to mention unspoken family rifts and having to watch your boyfriend turn into a 12-year-old again. However, getting on with his family doesn't have to be the straw that breaks the camel's back (and your relationship). All you need are some simple manoeuvres to get you through the ordeal of in-law bonding.

The mother from hell

Yes, she does exist, and your best bet is not to challenge her but to suck up, because she's going to criticise you anyway. Tell her that she made a great job of bringing up your boyfriend and ask her if she's got any tips. Don't, whatever you do, show her how much your boyfriend thinks of you – you know the truth and that's enough.

The holiday season cometh

Holidays are the worst time of the year to meet the in-laws, simply because this is when you have not only to be nice but also to spend 72 hours on the trot with them. Either make plans with your own family so that you can get away, or make sure you turn up at the end of the holiday, by which time they'll be sick of one another and you'll be the welcome new face.

Get an ally

To make family gatherings easier, find yourself an ally. It might be his sister, his brother or even an aunt – someone who can act as a buffer between you and his parents and ease family gatherings along. Having a family ally is also a good idea because it can give you an insight into your boyfriend's role in the family, and why his parents treat him the way they do.

Be a bitch on the inside

OK, so his dad's weird, his mum's rude and his sister's a psycho, but this is his family, meaning criticise them and all hell will break loose. Apart from the fact that all families are weird in their own way, openly bitching about his parents will be like a knife in his side. Let him do the criticising and nod in the appropriate places, and save your ranting for your friends.

Consider your prejudices

Being irritated with someone else's family often comes from prejudices you probably aren't admitting to. Do his parents annoy you because they're different from you? Do they hold different values, different morals, and different political views? All these things are fairly common and are easily solved with the realisation that you don't have to be best friends. Obviously it would be easier all round if you got on, but the fact is you don't have to be close to get by. If anything, maintaining a little distance can be good for your relationship, plus it's more genuine and gives his family a chance to see you the way he does.

Babe pointers

✦ **Don't try to ingratiate yourself** Otherwise known as: just be yourself. While it's tempting to be the ideal daughter-in-law, in the long run it won't do you any favours. Your boyfriend dated you for you yourself so he won't expect you to turn into the 'perfect' girlfriend for his parents.

✦ **Hold your tongue** So his father reads a rubbish paper and his mum has outdated ideas about the way her son should be looked after. Even if it causes every hair on your body to stand on end, just nod politely because you are never going to change them.

✦ **Don't make your boyfriend choose** It's tough for him too, and imagine how you'd feel if he asked the same of you. If the situation is really bad, just hit the main holiday such as Christmas and let him go visiting on his own the rest of the year.

✦ **Use your parents** Need to get out of things, dodge requests and favours but don't want to offend? Use your parents, it's a get-out clause that they can't argue with.

body

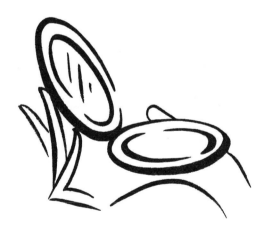

How to apply make-up like an expert

 Less is always more with make-up. As in: less overall volume of make-up and more time applying it. The aim of wearing make-up is not to achieve the same effect as cosmetic surgery (that is, give you a face even your mum wouldn't recognise) but to even up your skin tone and highlight the best of your features. This means none of us should be a slave to the latest make-up fashion. If you always dreamed of learning how to apply your make-up, here are the rules you should be observing.

Foundation

Don't commit the cardinal sin of foundation: testing it on your hand. To see if a colour works always try it on your jaw-line or face and then look at it in natural light. The shade that is right for your skin is one that should disappear into your skin.

Concealer

A girl's best make-up tool, but only if you use it correctly. Contrary to popular belief concealer should always come after your foundation so that it's not wiped off, and even though it's a shade lighter it should blend into your overall look. A yellow-based concealer is best, if you want to cancel out dark circles around your eyes.

Powder

Use powder not as a cover-up but to set foundation and absorb excess skin oil. Always apply it with a brush, but don't overdo it or you'll look 'dusty'.

Eyelashes and brows

Your eyebrows can either frame and highlight your eyes or lie there like giant caterpillars crawling across your face. The choice is yours, but if you do decide to tame them, it's worth opting for professional help. If not, pluck wayward hairs from underneath the brow with tweezers and smooth the rest with Vaseline.

For expert lashes, curl them before using mascara, as this makes them look fuller, then stroke the colour on your top lashes from roots to ends and go easy on the bottom row (it looks more natural).

Eyes

Going wrong with eyeshadow is common as people tend to forget that the aim is to see the eye, not the eyeshadow. Tip one is to use colours that belong to same family as the rest of your make-up. Then, to make your eyes look larger, go for a light colour. However, if your eyes are already full, go for soft darker shades instead. To stop the inevitable eyeshadow crease, put powder and foundation around your eye first.

Lips

Plump, sensual lips are a key player when you're flirting so it pays to know how to make the best of them. First prime them. A base coat of something clear keeps lips from drying out, especially if you're opting for a matt (non-glossy) colour. As for colour, don't be led by fashion – dark colours make your lips look thinner, whereas shades too light for your skin can make your make-up clash.

Babe pointers

+ **Vaseline** A good primer and excellent for fixing chapped lips and eyebrows that won't stay put.
+ **Eyelash curlers** To give your eyes that expert sparkle.
+ **Foundation sponge** Essential for even toning.
+ **Powder brush** Better than a sponge, as it won't dislodge all your hard work.
+ **Tweezers** Essential for brows.
+ **Cotton buds** Good application tools if you have no brushes.
+ **Tissues** Essential for blotting and placing under eyes when applying eyeshadow.
+ **A moisturiser with added sun protection factor (SPF)** Your make-up will lie better with this underneath.
+ **Make-up remover** Sleeping in your make-up won't kill you but it won't do much for your skin either.
+ **A mirror** You can't do much without one!

How to fix a hangover face

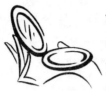

The weird thing about getting drunk is you can never quite recall the morning after the night before, until it starts happening all over again. If you've never woken up with a hangover it's worth knowing it's not a pretty sight. This is because the effects of over-drinking kill off your looks, thanks in most part to the dehydration effect, where water from your skin (along with blood supply) is directed away from your skin to more essential organs in your body. Add in the bad-sleep factor (being drunk means you sleep less effectively) and the fact that either you've eaten something large and greasy, or you're about to, and you're guaranteed to wake up looking and feeling as if you've landed in beauty hell. While the ideal solution is obviously not to drink, or better still to drink in moderation, the reality is it's best to know how to fix your face in order to face the day. Here's how.

Drink more water

This is the tip that just keeps on working. As water is the main thing that's lost from the body during an alcohol binge it pays to keep adding it back from the moment you get home. Drink half a litre (about one pint) before you go to bed and you'll wake feeling slightly better.

Massage your face

Rubbing your face will not only bring back the blood supply and leave you looking a bit healthier but also ease that tensed-up dehydration feeling in your skin. Using your forefingers, massage your face for ten minutes starting at the jawline and moving towards the ears and then the temple area. Next, press and rotate your fingers on the two points either side of your nose near to your eye sockets. Then move along your eyebrow line and forehead.

Slap on the moisturiser

Your skin is crying out for a drink so apply lashings of moisturiser to your face and balm to your lips the morning after and, if you're capable, the night before. A good face cream will attract water to your skin and help to hold it there.

Look after your eyes

A good tip for sore eyes is to keep your eye cream in the fridge so that it cools down your eyes when you rub it on (under and over the lid, not in your eye). De-bag the morning after with cold tea bags over the eyes and/or cucumber slices. For dry, smoke-ridden hangover eyes, try eye drops to refresh and rehydrate.

Avoid a face full of make-up

Tempting as it is to make yourself up to hide the effects of a hangover, it's worth noting that as blood is circulated away from the face, your make-up is likely to be a shade too dark so your best bet is a minimum effect – of powder, lip gloss and dark glasses.

Neutralise your breath

Alcohol also dries up your saliva leaving you prone to bad breath. The best cure is to chew sugar-free gum to activate saliva in your mouth. Chewing crystallised ginger does the same and also helps stop the accompanying morning-after nausea.

Babe pointers

+ **Concealer** is a girl's best morning-after friend.
+ **For dark spots** Use a thicker concealer or a light one mixed with a drop of your foundation.
+ **Blitz your dark circles** Concealer for dark circles needs to be opaque (not sheer) to cover the darker zones. Always use a brush or a sponge to make sure you're not caking it on and making it look worse.
+ **Kill two birds with one stone** For puffiness and circles under your eyes, blend your concealer with your eye cream. For skin, blend the concealer with a drop of foundation and moisturiser. Creamy concealers do the best all-round work for hangover faces.
+ **Detox your system** Think about what you eat. The sooner you detox your internal system, the sooner you'll look better externally. Think fresh fruit, plain food and not processed junk or a fried breakfast!

How to walk in heels

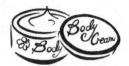 High heels – a girl's best friend. They make your legs look longer and sexier, help you to perfect an entrance and can even make you the envy of all the other girls in a room! Plus they tone the calf and thigh muscles and improve circulation in the legs. However, in order to walk in heels without tottering (the reason they call them totty shoes) you need strong stomach muscles to support you at the front and strong back muscles to support you at the rear.

The good news is if you can stand up straight in bare feet you can learn to work a room in heels. Here's how to do it.

Strengthen your stomach

If a night in heels makes you feel as if someone has kicked you in the back, your problem is having little or no stomach muscles. This means the muscles in your lower back have to support not only the back of you but the front as well. As heels throw you slightly off balance (the angle of the heel pushes your pelvis forwards), this instantly puts more pressure on your back. Solution: you need to build up your core strength (*see* How to get a flat stomach, page 144).

Remember: heels shouldn't hurt

If walking in heels makes you feel as if there are pins digging into the balls of your feet, you're not alone. The foot is the body's natural shock-absorber; tip your entire body weight from the whole of your foot and on to the ball of your foot and you'll feel pain. To stop the pain, slip your shoes off and massage the balls of your feet, then sit down (preferably with your legs up) for ten minutes to allow the circulation back. Then, to stand tall, keep your feet hip-width apart (your hips are smaller than you think) and imagine there is a string pulling you up from the centre of your head.

Walk the walk

Now you can stand in high heels, all that's left is to walk confidently in them. This takes practice, so when you have an event you want to make an impact at the trick is to start wearing in your shoes two weeks beforehand. To get used to standing, sitting, bending and moving in heels, wear them when you do the housework. It sounds pervy, but it works. Next, watch how the professionals do it. Models get it right because they walk confidently in heels, slightly swinging their hips to gain momentum. If sashaying into a room isn't your thing, be sure to walk confidently (practise with a book on your head). Meaning don't teeter along with your bottom out, or stomp, because it's not sexy and you'd look better in flats.

Babe pointers

+ **Opt for height and width**
  Especially if you've never worn high heels before, because the wider the width of the heel the more stable you'll be (a bigger surface area for your weight to balance on).

+ **Cheat with a wedge** With a wedge heel you can go higher but still feel as if you're walking on relatively flat heels. This is because the wedge decreases the angle of the heel along the sole of your foot, meaning your foot won't have to arch too much.
+ **Pick a shoe/boot with a strap or laces** Tying a high heel to your leg can give you more stability when you're walking, as your foot is secure. Remember: if a shoe's too high when you're in a shop, it's too high to buy.
+ **Alternate your shoes** Alternating between high and low heels enables your physique to adapt and benefit. Low heels about 2.5cm (1in) in height are good for the front and back of the foot, and help reduce tension in the tendons and ligaments around the foot.
+ **How to dance** Less is more when dancing in heels. The trick is to keep your feet still, and grind and move your upper body and hips – then, bingo! you're dancing.

How to survive a bad-hair day

Bad-hair days are the same as those look-in-the-mirror-and-want-to-go-back-to-bed days. They're the days when your hair basically gives you a clear indication that today is not going to be a good day no matter what you do. Whether it's because your roots are coming through, a couple of grey strands have appeared, or you have no discernible style, it looks like nothing could save you.

Feeling horrible about yourself when your hair looks horrible is relatively common, and has much to do with the way we view ourselves. Most of us look in a mirror and focus on our head-to-neck region; if your hair (which, let's face it, tends to be the largest mass on and around your face) looks strange, it's natural to assume that now your whole face does as well. Ridiculous, but true for most of us. While the solution lies in dealing with your hair (see below) it's also worth noting that to keep your hair at its healthiest and happiest, it really helps if you can actually feel happy too. Here's how to get your hair to behave.

Product overload
If you're regularly running gel, mousse, spray and fix-it holds through your hair, it's worth noting that a fast shampoo (even a daily one) won't help. To rid hair of product build-up you need to shampoo thoroughly with a good shampoo. A dollop the size of a small circle is all you should need.

Blast your hair with cold air
Cold air pointed at the roots of your hair will lift the hair. To lift fine or thinning hair, also consider a colour, which will plump up the cuticle and improve the condition.

Figure out the time of the month
PMS days and period days tend to affect

the way your hair looks and feels, and more often than not are the real reason behind bad-hair days. This is all down to fluctuating hormones in the body, so don't do anything radical until your period is near its end then think cut, style, and maybe even colour.

Dry your hair properly

Don't spend ages washing your hair and then try to dry it at 100 mph. Apart from turning your head into a frizz ball, it will dry out your hair. To dry hair more efficiently, wait before you blow-dry. Hair that's 80 per cent dry before blasting will end up less damaged.

See a hairdresser

Like getting your car an MOT, it's essential to get hair seen by an expert on a regular basis. Bad-hair days are usually indicative of the fact that you need a haircut or at least an MOT. A good hairdresser will not only advise you on the products you're using but also tell you the exact condition of your hair and what to do about it.

Babe pointers

+ **Frizzy hair** The best way to deal with frizzy, curly hair is to shampoo not every day but every other day, so you don't wash the oil out of the hair. Then, before conditioning, dry off your hair using a towel so that you don't dilute the conditioner; keep it on for two minutes and wash off.

+ **Greasy hair** The best way to avoid a greasy scalp is to wash your hair every day with a mild shampoo and be sure not to load up on hair products. If your hair has suddenly become greasy, check to see that it isn't a new shampoo or product that's making it lank.

+ **Dry hair is a sign your hair is dying for a drink** To hydrate it feed it more conditioner, preferably one that you can leave in, and don't blitz your hair with a dryer.

+ **Limp hair** When hair goes limp, products are to blame. Help yourself – either switch to a light conditioner or skip them all together.

+ **If all else fails wear a hat** This one is guaranteed to work!

How to look better naked

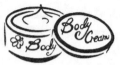 If you think this one's an impossibility – then either you've got body-dysmorphic syndrome or you need a huge self-esteem boost. Looking better naked is simply about forgetting your flaws and dumping your insecurities about lumps, bumps and odd bits. It's also about being proud to get naked and bare all if not for the sake of your confidence then for the sake of your sex life (ask any man – there's nothing sexier than a woman who's OK with her body). Exercise and diet aside, there is many a thing you can do to improve the look and feel of your skin. Here's what to try.

Cellulite busting

This is the stuff that resembles dimply, orange peel, appears mainly on the thighs and bottom and affects around 85 per cent of us. The good news is you can beat it, and without paying out for expensive creams or downing gallons of water.

Reducing the level of fat in the blood is key to getting rid of cellulite. Aim for more exercise and foods rich in Omega 3 fatty acids (EFAs), found in oily fish and nuts. Not only do these regulate the speed at which fat is released into the body but research shows they also have a definite anti-cellulite effect.

Pedicures

Don't forget your feet. Sexy feet go far in helping you to look better naked, so think of a foot 'facial'. Whereas it's possible to do a DIY job, it always pays to see a chiropodist who can remove corns and thickened skin quickly and give you a good base to work from. To do it at home you will need a pumice stone, thick skin cream and a nail-buffer. Always work on your feet after they have been soaking for ten minutes, so nails and skin are soft.

Body hair

To zap or not to zap is a personal issue, but if you hate the look of body hair the best way to get rid of it is to wax or shave.

Never use a razor on dry skin unless

you want to go for a hacked-up look, and while it's fine to shave under arms, shaving thighs and bikini line can lead to a nasty scratchy feeling when the hair grows back (not sexy). For a home bikini wax, preparation is the key:

Don't have a hot bath or sunbathe before going for a wax, as when your skin is hot the wax heats up, which can lead to potential scars and more pain when the strip is peeled off. Also don't let things overgrow, as this means more waxing, more pain, and post-wax soreness. For the actual wax, you don't have to be a contortionist. Sit on a stool or the edge of a bath, sit as far back as you can and spread your legs. Trim hair to 5mm (¼in) first and dust talc on to your legs to stop the wax from sticking. Pull skin taut, press on a cloth strip and pull in the direction of growth.

Babe pointers

+ **Get real** Specifically about your perceived flaws, otherwise you will spend your life hating yourself and your body. Remember: either change the bits you don't like (through diet and exercise) or accept them and learn to enjoy what you have.

+ **Get used to seeing yourself naked** Bare bodies can be a shock if you never look at what you've got. Spend at least five minutes a day walking around naked to get used to the look and feel of your body. The more you do this and the more you look at yourself naked, the nicer your body will look to you.

+ **Sneak looks at other people** Not a cue to become a peeping Tom, but more a wake-up call to see that we're all made strangely. Only models in magazines look 'perfect'; on the whole the rest of us are thankfully all too long/short/fat/skinny, and so on.

+ **Make the best of what you've got** We all have areas of our body that are good. Accentuate the positive

How to get a flat stomach

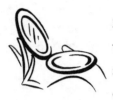

Sick of sucking in your tummy? Fed up with seeing stomach overhang? Well, if you want to transform yourself from belly-babe to Über-babe the good news is you can. A flat stomach, believe it or not, is not hard to achieve, and the reason most of us don't display a toned midriff is a combination of the five following elements: the kind of food we eat, the fluids we consume, bad posture, excess body fat and the wrong kind of stomach exercises. Meaning if you've been doing 100 sit-ups a day, eating doughnuts and washing it down with fizzy pop, your stomach will be more concertina-shaped than flat. Here's how to reverse the look.

Lose weight

You're never going to see a washboard tummy if it's covered in a layer of fat, which is why your first objective should be to eat healthily and do at least 20 minutes of aerobic exercise four to five times a week for fat-burning.

Do specific exercises

Your first step should be to veto the traditional sit-up/crunch, as this won't help you get a flat stomach because it engages the wrong muscles. The good news is that the following exercises will work on the right muscles:

The bicycle

Lie on the floor with your lower back pressed into the ground. Put your hands behind your head as you lift it off the ground. Now move your legs to a 45-degree angle and begin a bicycling motion, while touching your left elbow to your right knee, and your right elbow to your left knee. Do three sets of ten.

Knee raises

Sit on the edge of a stable chair, knees bent, and feet flat on the floor; hold on to the sides of the chair for support. Tighten your tummy to support your back and lift your feet several inches off the floor.

Now, in a steady movement, pull your knees in towards your chest and pull your upper body forward. Lower your feet to their original position, and repeat. Do three sets of ten.

Build core strength

For those who can't find good posture easily, start working your deep postural muscles, which run around the body like a corset. Building these muscles creates what's known as core stability to help you look taller, and your stomach flatter. Try this for five minutes three times a day:

Breathe in, place your hand on your bellybutton and, on the out breath, pull your stomach and lower abdominals in. Imagine your bellybutton being pulled back towards your spine. Hold for three counts and repeat.

Eat proper food

For swift results you need to beat the fat and the bloat. Retaining water and having gas in your stomach will sabotage your chances of getting a flat look. If you suffer from stomach bloating, avoid eating too many starchy carbohydrates; choose lean meats, vegetables, fruits and salads; and avoid processed foods.

Babe pointers

+ **Drink more water** Aim for about eight to ten glasses every day. Not drinking enough is bad news for the digestive system especially if you load up with coffee, alcohol, tea and fizzy drinks, which all lead to stomach bloating.
+ **Eat little and often** So your body doesn't crave quick fixes, such as chocolate, which can lead to weight gain.
+ **Cut out the fat** That's the fat-inducing refined carbohydrates and sugars (cakes and biscuits to you and me!) by not buying ready-made meals and fast food.
+ **Work your stomach** Try to tense your stomach muscles whenever you remember to and for as long as you can. This will help tone up your muscles and burn calories.
+ **Be realistic** Six-pack stomachs tend to occur only in very thin or athletic people as a result of very low body fat. Aim for less of a stomach rather than hoping to achieve a model-like one.

How to get rid of batwing arms

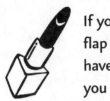

If your batwings jiggle and flap long after your arms have stopped moving and you dread the return of summer because of short-sleeved tops, you've come to the right section. But exercise alone won't get you there. If you exercise and don't change your diet, all that will happen is your arms will get bigger as well as firmer.

Lifting weights is the ideal road to go down. This is because you need to work the biceps and triceps in your arms in order to tone up. Muscles grow in strength and leanness by an overloading of the muscle fibres. Your arms then look leaner because muscle takes up three times less space than fat.

Shadow boxing

This is where you continuously punch the air for 30 seconds non-stop (think *Rocky*). For the first ten seconds it feels like you're doing nothing and then muscle fatigue sets in. Repeat on both arms and then do the whole set again when you have completed the exercises below.

Lateral raise

This helps tone and shape your shoulders and lats (muscles under your armpits). Stand up straight with your feet hip-width apart, shoulders pulled down (imagine your shoulder blades sliding down your back) and stomach pulled in. Now, with weights (2kg/4½lb) in your hands and your elbows slightly bent, raise the weights out to the sides until your hands are level with your shoulders with your palms facing the floor. Hold for a second and repeat. Do three sets of 15.

Close-grip press-up

Perfect for instant toning of the chest and the arms. Start by lying face down and placing your hands directly under your shoulders (palms facing forwards). Keeping your stomach pulled in, and your body straight (or resting on your knees if you're a complete beginner), bend your arms to 90 degrees, then push yourself back up and start again. The trick is to pull down under your arms to support your body while supporting your back with your stomach muscles. Build to three sets of 12 repetitions.

Triceps dips

The triceps is the underused muscle on the underside of your arm, so it pays to do lots of these. Sit on the edge of a sturdy chair and place your hands either side of your bottom. Hold on to the edge of the chair. Your legs should be hip-width apart and bent to 90 degrees. Start by moving your bottom forwards off the chair then lower your bottom towards the floor by bending your arms, and then rise up by pushing up with your arms. Do three sets of 10–15 repetitions. To make the exercise more challenging, straighten your legs (move them further away from your body).

Bicep curls

For those sexy upper-arm muscle bumps, stand up straight with your feet hip-width apart, shoulders back and stomach pulled in. Hold a weight in each hand (3kg/6½lb), with your arms straight and your hands facing upwards. Now bend your elbows (keeping them tucked in) and curl the weight towards your

shoulders (keeping your upper body still). Hold for a second and slowly lower all the way down again (do the whole range of movement so you don't shorten the muscle). Do three sets of 10–15 repetitions.

Babe pointers

+ **Do more sport** Arms get flabby because they are underused, so consider trying tennis, badminton, squash and even Boxercise lessons.
+ **Work more than your arms** Don't forget to work your shoulders, back and chest too – these all add to perfect arms.
+ **Be realistic** It's tempting to lust after the shape of someone else's arms, but while you can perfect your own look it's virtually impossible to get the arms of someone with a different body shape to yours.
+ **Think posture** It won't make your arms firm, but standing upright, shoulders back, stomach in and head held high will instantly make you look seven pounds thinner.

How to lose weight

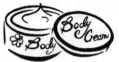 Life is different at 25 from at 35, which is why a chocolate croissant goes from your mouth to your waist far more quickly as you get older than it used to do. The culprit here (apart from the amount you eat) is your metabolism – this is the way your body burns calories. While some lucky souls have a speedy metabolic rate, which allows them to eat a pint of Häagen-Dazs and never gain a pound, most of us will experience a natural 5 to 10 per cent slowing-down in our metabolic rate every decade. This translates as burning 100 fewer calories a day at 35 than we did at 25, which equals a weight gain of around a pound a year!

To lose weight the equation is simple: eat less and do more. It doesn't matter if you're big-boned, have a predisposition to gaining weight, have tried every diet in the book, or have a slow metabolism – if you follow the above you will lose weight. If you want to lose excess pounds here's what you need to do.

Forget fad diets

These diets may work in the short run but they are not designed to keep the weight off. Weight loss should be achieved at two pounds a week (unless you have a lot to lose) otherwise you're going to regain it. Never trust a fad diet that promises more than this, or that tells you to eat only one type of food, or if it sounds too good to be true.

Keep it simple

Diets don't have to be complicated to work. Eat more fruit and vegetables (five portions a day if possible), choose lean meat and fish, grill and bake your food rather than frying it and cut back on sugar-laden foods, such as processed meals, alcohol, cakes, biscuits and chocolate.

Exercise

Sorry, but if you want to lose weight you've got to do some exercise, as it will speed up your metabolism. Also, toned muscle tissue has a much higher metabolic rate than fat, meaning you will burn more calories and so you'll see results more quickly.

Eat more food

Research shows that nearly 70 per cent of us regularly miss a meal every day. This is bad news if you're trying to lose weight, because after four hours without food the body will suppress its ability to burn calories in order to conserve energy. What most people don't realise is that your metabolism rises when you eat, because the body needs to burn energy for digesting and absorbing food. Meaning you have to eat to lose weight.

Babe pointers

+ **Eat breakfast** Your mother was right: breakfast is the most important meal of the day, especially as far as weight loss is concerned. This is because our metabolism naturally slows down when we sleep and won't rev up until we eat again.

+ **Pump iron** Lift weights and you won't beef up but you'll look smaller, as muscle takes up three times less space than fat. Even better news is that one pound of lean muscle burns nine times more calories than a pound of fat.

+ **Eat protein** Focus on protein to stoke your fat-burning fires. Not only is it harder to digest and so uses 20–30 per cent more energy for digestion (an extra 150 to 200 calories a day) but it also forces your metabolic rate upwards.

+ **Go to bed earlier** A study from the University of Chicago shows that getting less than five hours sleep a night leads to the body's over-producing insulin, which in turn promotes fat storage.

How to get the body you want

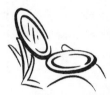

Getting the body you want isn't so much to do with eating celery for life and spending all your spare time at the gym. It's more about that old favourite: getting real. Roughly translated this means the body you want may not be the body you can have! The truth is most of us have unrealistic expectations about our bodies and lust after bodies that generally are out of our scope – think pop stars, glamour models and long-legged actresses. Women in the public eye are not representative of the general population, as most have been preened, surgically enhanced and digitally remastered to look so fabulous. Those who haven't gone down that path tend to have trainers, chefs, stylists and make-up artists on hand 24/7 to help them look so natural; then there are those who are just genetically blessed to have a body type that most of us will never get to.

This doesn't mean give up and eat doughnuts for ever, but instead focus on a body goal that you can actually achieve so that: (1) you won't get disheartened and give up; (2) you won't become obsessed and bore everyone; and (3) you will eventually be happy with the outcome. Set your goal too high or make it too unbelievable, and even if you reach your target weight and have everyone telling you that you look gorgeous, you will still feel that you've failed.

What's your true shape?

Look at your family. If everyone in your family is more weeble-shaped than Kate Moss-shaped, then the chances are that while you can be slim, you're never going to parade down a Paris catwalk. Some people are naturally lean with long legs and arms, others are prone to the athletic, strong look, and others still have a curvy body and are also likely to be of average height or less. Of course, you can also be a mix of all of the above but it can help to know what body type you're working with, in order to make sure you're not trying to turn an Amazonian look into a teeny-tiny girl look.

Set small goals

Once you've pinpointed the shape you're working with, be sure to set small goals, as no one keeps up any exercise or healthy eating plan if their goals are too high. This means don't aim to work out five days a week if you're currently averaging five times a year. Be clear with yourself. If you want to get in shape, you have to work at it consistently.

Motivate yourself

Three months is a good deadline for your end goal, which could be a holiday, a wedding or a special event. Within this time you should have three process goals. Goal one: go to the gym twice a week; goal two: eat sensibly and control your portions; and goal three: limit alcohol and junk food when you go out.

Babe pointers

✦ **Find a realistic role model** This should be someone whose body shape is like yours. Ask your mum or best friend for an honest opinion as to whether you're being realistic or not.

✦ **Work out why you want to look a certain way** Is it because you're hoping it will bring you a lifestyle/ boyfriend/love? If so, it's worth knowing that the people most successful at reaching their body goals get there because they are doing it for health and self-esteem reasons only.

✦ **Avoid quick fixes** As tempting as it is to go down a fad-diet-and-over-training route, for long-term success that sticks opt for a healthy diet with a little bit of what you fancy and a more active life with exercise.

✦ **Detox for a week** One week of eating well, with no drinking, no sugar, no alcohol, lots of sleep and three sessions of working out gently. This will give you a good weight loss that will psychologically boost your motivation and get you closer to the body you can have.

confidence

· ·

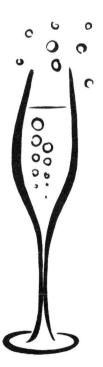

How to make small talk

Small talk, otherwise known as mindless chatter, instantly forgettable conversation and space fillers, is not as easy as most people think. Do it right and you can actually have a fairly enjoyable conversation about cleaning the oven; do it wrong and you'll end up prattling away about developing world politics and blindly putting your foot in it. Want to be the queen of nothing speak? Here's how.

It's not what you talk about

It's actually about how interesting you make your subject. In general, the most obvious small-talk subject is the weather. Most people will quite happily discuss how much rain there's been, how little sun and how grey the sky is for hours if need be. However, if climate changes aren't your thing, then simply choose any subject but give it a frame of reference, such as 'I hate housework but really don't think this bar could do with a clean? Think of the dust mites.' Giving the person you're chatting to the chance to reply with a comment about cleaning, allergies, and/or the hostess's domestic skills.

Don't get personal

Small talk is not really about discovering anything other than someone's name, because it's not about sharing intimacies or building a friendship. By the time you start with small talk you already know that you're never going to see this person again. They won't be at your wedding, you don't know anyone who knows them and really they're quite dull – so what's the point? Well, apart from being polite, the point is to pass the time and you may as well do it pleasurably. If you're never going to see them again this is your chance to embellish your life (that is, lie a little), show off, make jokes your friends wouldn't laugh at, and most of all test how good your social conversation skills are on strangers.

Don't make a speech

A soliloquy is not small talk. The poor person who just got lumbered with you isn't interested in what you think of the Third World debt, why you became an accountant and the names of your three cats. Just entertain each other by talking about nothing. Small-talk topics include TV, your immediate environment, the latest film you saw, something one of you is wearing, and even how you came to be talking to each other. It doesn't require effort, argument or even a huge amount of energy, and if it does, you're not making small talk.

When in doubt

Just interview the person. Imagine you're a journalist and go down the who, what, where and how route. People mostly love to talk about themselves, so you'll have not only a willing chatter but also a chance to look interested and interesting to everyone around you. If, however, you're unlucky enough to be with Monosyllabic Man, turn the tables on him, ignore the point above and bore him until he goes away.

Babe pointers

✦ **Small talk, as in the word 'small'** 'Inconsequential talk' would be a better, although longer, way of describing small talk, which means if you feel stuck for how to do it just observe 85 per cent of the conversations around you.

✦ **If you hate it, keep it brief** Studies show that women use small talk as a way to discover information, and men use it as a way to pass the time. If you truly loathe it, keep it brief, and make an excuse to walk away.

✦ **Have an opinion** It's OK to have an opinion with small talk, in fact it's often better if you do as it spices the chat up.

✦ **Don't judge people on their chat** In my time I have had whole conversations about vacuum cleaners, toilet paper and the many uses of make-up concealer! Does it make me exceedingly strange? Maybe, but it doesn't tell you anything about me – apart from perhaps I have too much spare time on my hands.

How to boost your confidence

You may not be shy, quiet or even timid, but everyone, no matter how confident, can do with an 'I'm great really' boost now and again. If you're feeling flat, fed up and just downright blah, here's how to boost your confidence and look on the brighter side of life.

Support others
You'll be amazed at how giving others confidence and a sense of achievement can make you feel great about yourself and your own achievements. Dish out some compliments, tell people how they make you feel and give someone a supportive shoulder to lean on. Better still take up mentoring, and mentor a child – local charities, local schools and national organisations all run these schemes.

Do something challenging
Scuba dive, climb a mountain, aim to run a marathon by next year, take up a sport you've never considered, learn a language – the list is endless. Challenging things force us to move off our square of security and try things we never thought we were capable of. Becoming a physical person when you thought you weren't, or an academic one when you were sure you didn't have it in you, will not only boost your confidence but also help change your whole perception of yourself.

Change your look
A change is as good as a rest, and nothing will make you more confident than either changing your look or improving upon it. Cut your hair; have it straightened/curled/dyed; change your make-up; throw away your wardrobe and go for a totally new look. You don't have to be stuck in a rut just because everyone thinks you're the denim girl, or assumes you always have to go glam.

Don't be defined by other people's labels
Having friends who have known you for years is wonderful, but not if they're always determined to see you as Miss

Sensible or Miss No Hoper. Make your own labels and challenge people's perspective of you. So what if you don't look the type to sky-dive off mountains – you can be anyone you want to be, anytime you choose to be.

Give yourself a sense of achievement

Instead of remembering all the things that have gone wrong in your life, or why you're single/bored/unfit/stuck in a job, think about all the good things you've done – where you've been, what you've achieved and are proud of – and then give yourself a pat on the back. Now list all the things you're good at, such as being a good friend, having a good sense of humour, cooking, running, even putting an outfit together. Remember: anything and everything counts when it comes to confidence-boosting. It's not being bigheaded, it's all about appreciating your worth.

Babe pointers

+ **Ask around for feelgood comments** Tell your friends you're feeling blue and ask them for a confidence boost. There's nothing wrong in asking for compliments and reassurance when you're feeling flat.
+ **Look at the past** And consider how you've changed for the better in terms of being a good friend/girlfriend/ daughter. How confident are you now compared to when you were younger? What have you improved on/conquered and made good?
+ **Focus on moving forwards** This is the direction you should always be moving in. What's your game plan for the next six months? What do you hope to do or learn? Where do you wish to go? Knowing where you're heading can give you a surge of confidence about the future.
+ **Be grateful** This is a huge confidence-booster. Look at all the fabulous things in your life and list them in a gratitude book. How lucky are you? What do you have to be proud and confident about?

How to beat shyness

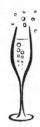 If you're shy, you'll know the horror of having to walk into a room alone, speaking on the phone to someone you don't know, or even starting to make small talk to people at parties. Shyness can often feel like a kind of torture and a curse – and if you don't conquer it, it can affect everything from your career chances to your love life. Here's how to work your way through it.

Focus outward

Shyness is a form of self-consciousness and is linked to low self-esteem. It basically means that when you meet someone new, or even walk into a shop, you feel crippled by a sense of not knowing what to say and assume right off that everyone is thinking the worst of you. If you want to deal with it, the first thing to do is to shine that spotlight off you and on to what you're looking at. Focus outwardly not internally, and instead of thinking, 'My God, what does this person think of me?' say to yourself, 'This person seems nice – what do I want to know about them?'

Speak up

Shyness often comes across as unfriendliness, so if you're feeling timid, just smile – it says a lot more than you think. Next, practise speaking up for yourself. As with anything that's hard, practice takes the rough edges off it. Firstly your opinion is worth as much as anyone else's, and secondly you're not going to look stupid (and, really, so what if you do?). Take small steps first. Ask for something in a shop, say something at a meeting, and introduce yourself to someone at a party. Remember: no one is expecting you to be funny, clever or razor sharp – just be friendly.

Take yourself out of your comfort zone

It's probably nice and safe where you are – you know your friends and you're happy where you work. However, to beat shyness you have to push the boundaries of your world regularly. Do something you're afraid of every day, even if it's talking to the postman on Monday, and expressing an opinion on Tuesday. Building up your courage like this will not only lessen your shyness, but also help you to see that the reality never lives up to the fear in your head.

Shyness is learnt behaviour

While we're not all born extroverts, shyness does tend to come from learnt behaviour, which is good news because it means you can unlearn it. Work out what you're getting from being shy (remember none of us ever does anything painful that doesn't give us a positive outcome). Does it get you attention? Does it help you to feel safe? Do you use it as a good excuse to stop trying?

To change, think about all the things that won't happen in your life if you remain shy: all the things you won't experience; the people you won't meet; and the things you will miss out on. It's depressing and painful (or it should be) but if you recall this list every time shyness holds you back, it will propel you forwards to break your pattern of shyness.

Babe pointers

✦ **We're all worried about ourselves** Most people are just adept at not showing it. And the reality is no one's looking at you, because everyone's too busy worrying about themselves.

✦ **Fake it to make it** Looking confident when you don't feel it is the key to social situations. Hold your head up, throw your shoulders back and walk tall to create a positive impression on others.

✦ **Make eye contact** Not looking at someone when you speak or while he or she is talking often comes across as lack of interest. Maintain their gaze for at least three seconds before you look away, and when they are talking you should be looking at them for about 80 per cent of the time.

✦ **Ask your friends for tips** Most people feel shy in certain situations. Ask your friends for their anti-shyness tips and see if they work for you. Talking about it takes away the pressure of feeling all alone in this.

How to say hard things

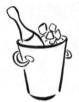

Being a straight talker is hard: it's tough to hear and tell the truth, and in reality no one wants to be the tough guy who has to lay it on the line. Sadly, in life tough things have to be said. People have to be reprimanded at work, partners have to be dumped, friends have to be told where to get off and rude shop girls have to be told, well, that they're being rude. If you find it hard to stand up for yourself, here's how to find your tough-love voice.

Are you sure you're right?

This is an ideal place to start if you're considering saying something hard to someone. The problem with smart people is (and let's face it we all consider ourselves to be smart) that we all think we're right. If you're unsure about the situation, ask the opinion of an outsider and find out if your stance is valid. Then before you say anything ask yourself, 'Is it worth it?' Meaning is this something that needs to done or something you feel like doing? Nine times out of ten it needs to be done, but it's always worth asking anyway.

Be fair

Going for their Achilles heel, such as listing everything that annoys you about them, and saying that X and Y also agree with you are not fair tactics. Not only does it put the person immediately on the defensive but also it detracts from your message. The key is to be both forceful and gentle. Say what you think, even if you think it makes you unpopular, but say it in a way that's not aggressive and antagonistic.

Get to the point

People know when bad news is coming, and anyone who knows you will know when you're struggling to say something hard. Don't torment them and make it worse for yourself by making excuses for what you're about to say. Make your point and then listen to the response. If you don't think they are going to understand, use a metaphor that works for them. For example, if they are into music or sport, make a comparison with something you know they'll be able to grasp. Above everything, be absolutely clear, especially if you're firing someone, breaking up with someone, or telling someone a friendship is over. Water down what you're saying and you'll think you've said one thing, and they will think they've heard another.

Be aware you could be wrong

We're all myopic to some degree – we see things only from our own perspective. The key is to try to see others as they see themselves so you can work out where they are coming from. The chances are up until this point they had no idea you were about to say what you just said, so be kind.

Babe pointers

✦ **Your mother was right** Treat people the way you expect to be treated. That is to say, be fair, be clear and be nice. Hearing hard things hurts, and your being nasty on top just turns that knife even further and does your cause no good.

✦ **Keep it short** After saying your piece, don't enter into endless discussion about it. If it was well thought out, it is likely that was what you wanted to say. Of course the other person will want to change your mind – don't let them.

✦ **Say it once, twice at the most** Repeating your statement over and over looks like you're unsure about yourself. It looks more confident to say it once with conviction and then keep quiet.

✦ **Make sure you tell people what you want** Just listing your grievances is one thing, but you need always to round it off with a conclusion. What do you want them to do (leave? change? apologise?) and what do you think will make things better?

How to hear hard things

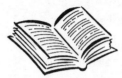 OK, so nobody's perfect, but that's not the ideal response when a lover's just told you you're a nightmare when you're drunk/sober/breathing, and so on. While it's never nice to hear that people have actually noticed we are less than perfect, it's worth noting that it's going to happen, and more than once in a lifetime. Here's how to hear and respond if someone's just handed you a personal critique.

Accept that your first response will be denial

Mixed with a hearty dose of irritation and a smattering of defensiveness. Hearing criticism, no matter how constructive, is painful because it makes us feel vulnerable and pathetic. So the first rule is to stop and listen to what's being said. Are they right? Maybe. Do you deserve to hear this? Maybe not! However, it's been said, so calm down and face it.

Hold the insults

You're not five years old so avoid the temptation to say, 'Yeah, but you smell/behave worse than me/act like that too.' All this kind of response will do is reinforce the person's view and make you feel idiotic and even more defensive. Also, bear in mind there is no truly easy way to tell someone something hard, which means it's taken a lot of personal courage for this person to look you in the eye and tell you this. Meaning this person is serious and you need to hear what's being said.

Take responsibility

But only for the parts you agree with. A boyfriend tells you it hurts when you spend all night talking to your friends and ignoring him. Apologise for hurting him (after all, your behaviour did), reassure him that it won't happen again and then explain why it might have happened. This way he will feel heard by you, before you start trying to wriggle out of it. Of course, there will be times when you don't feel what's been said is your responsibility, and that's fair enough, but ensure you listen and think before you come to that conclusion.

Don't ignore what's been said

It's tempting to put what's been said down to someone's bad day, or a PMS mood, but avoid this at all costs. Whether their motives are dodgy or not, you need to consider what's been said and what you're going to do about it. If you don't agree, this needs to be discussed. If you agree, this needs to be said. If you're not bothered, you haven't listened to what's been said, and if you're angry you need to admit it.

If you're too hurt to go on — say so

Just as people have the right to say hard things to you, you have the right to walk away, leave and generally cut yourself off if you don't like what's being said. However, be clear about your reasons and what you're doing. Remember that a little discomfort now will spare you the pain of more discussion later.

Babe pointers

+ **Learn something from this** Even if it's to choose your friends/lovers and work more carefully. On the whole, when hard things are said, there are valuable lessons you can learn about how you conduct yourself and what others find acceptable or not.

+ **Don't take on someone else's neuroses** A friend who is always blaming you for her life, her feelings and her misery is no friend. While we all do our best not to hurt the feelings of others, some people choose to be hurt in spite of our efforts. Weed them out.

+ **Have boundaries** Yes, people are allowed to say hard things to you but they are not allowed to get personal for no reason, bully you, or try to get you to conform to their ideals because they think they are right.

+ **Say, 'I don't agree' if you don't agree** It's powerful, it gets the point home and it isn't aggressive. If they then get hysterical, you will have the upper hand and the right simply to walk away.

How to deal with rude people

The world is full of rude people. Waiters who look through you, people who walk into you on the street, idiots who steal your parking spaces, shop assistants who can't be bothered to help ... the list is endless and horribly frustrating simply because it leaves us feeling belittled, maddened and somehow despised for no reason whatsoever. If you're constantly thinking, 'I'm a good person, I didn't deserve that,' here's how to deal with the rudest of the rude.

Don't take it personally

They are probably having a bad day, or maybe they just got dumped, or perhaps it's a hormonal surge. Whatever their excuse, it wasn't a personal and intimate attack on you, based on any knowledge of you. *However*, this doesn't mean you have to: (1) take it; (2) forgive it; or (3) ignore it. To get over it, you need to deal with it and take action immediately. The best road is to say, 'Excuse me but you're being very rude,' and look at them sternly (not aggressively).

Be sure what you want

It helps to know how this situation could be rectified in your favour. Are you looking for an apology, compensation or just plain acknowledgement that this isn't a way to behave? In most cases people are shocked into apologising immediately (or stunned into silence).

If you don't get the response you desire and you're in a shop/calling a utility company, ask for a more senior person or a customer services number. Be clear and consistent about what happened and what would make it better for you.

Choose your battles wisely

There are some levels of rude behaviour not worth tackling on your own and these include rudeness from drunken groups of people, people who cut you up on the road, and the clearly insane. All could result in more than hurt feelings, so a better option is to take a deep breath and let it go (in the US alone 15,000 people were injured in road-rage incidents in 2003).

Don't relive the moment over and over

Yes, you want to tell a friend about your moment of outrage, but retell the story ten times in a day and all you're doing is reliving the frustration and upset again and again and again. The rude person has probably already forgotten what he/she said or did, so why are you giving them more time and attention than they deserve?

Practise standing up for yourself

Not just when people have been rude but in your everyday life when people take you for granted, shut a door in your face, try to queue-push or generally try to get you to say 'Yes' when you've already said 'No'. Small successes with confronting minor uncomfortable situations help you to find the courage and confidence to tackle the larger and more hurtful ones.

Babe pointers

+ **Think past the initial embarrassment** Confrontation is hard, but take a deep breath and you can do it, and it's not as hard as spending the whole day feeling upset and unsettled. Plus it's not as embarrassing to do as you may think.

+ **Get your timing right** Yelling at the waiter before he's brought your meal out is probably a bad idea, as is screaming at a shop assistant before she goes off to check the stock room. Likewise, with friends and partners, avoid birthdays and seasonal celebrations for tough talking.

+ **Drop hints** Make subtle and not so subtle hints before you do the tough talking. This should force the person to ask what's up or simply give them the idea that it's time to shape up.

+ **Check who's being rude** Stooping to the rude level of someone else rarely makes you feel better or helps you to keep the moral high ground. As tempting as it is to shout back, restrain yourself, maintain your dignity and take heed of the above.

How to influence others

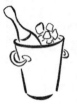

No, this is not the part where I tell you how to hypnotise others, make them bend to your will, or sign over their money and assets. It's the part where I try to persuade you to look at how to get what you want by influencing others. Hopefully you're not a wannabe dictator rubbing your hands in glee at the very thought of all that power, but someone who wants to know how to use their personality traits and skills for the best. If so, here's how to do it.

Be nice

It sounds ridiculous, but people like people who are, well, likeable. It makes them trust you, find similarities with you and want to build a rapport with you. This is the key to being influential, as rapport means you have persuaded someone that you not only think alike but also have each other's best interests at heart. Of course, it's more than being Mr Nice Guy, and has plenty to do with your body language and voice. Mirror them (not obviously) by mimicking their voice patterns and language use, and they'll feel a bond with you and won't even know why.

Speak with authority

It's amazing what you can get away with if you speak as if you know what you're talking about. This isn't an invitation to bluff your way into things, but a chance to get your authentic opinions heard. Spend a day listening to people and see what techniques they use to get you to believe them. It's those who don't look for constant reassurance when they speak, and speak with gravity, who are the ones whom others are most likely to listen to and believe.

Evoke emotion

You think it would be plain hard facts that persuade others to do things, but studies show that the majority of our decisions are based on our emotions. If you want someone to like you, listen to you and take your side, use emotions to get them there. If you can get them to associate you with feelgood emotions, they'll feel more associated with you. One way to do this is to get them to talk about happy events, or better still make them laugh and feel good. Try complimenting them (but honesty counts, as the second they think you're faking you will have lost them). Be funny and, better still, show them a good time so they will associate you with the happier things in life.

Make people feel special

Most people go through life not feeling valued or listened to. If you can get someone to feel both, not only will they feel linked to you for life but also they will trust you. Ways to do this are simple: let them know that you hear what they are saying; remember personal facts about them so they feel that you care; and, finally, don't take advantage of them. Manage all that and you've pretty much got them leading your cheerleading squad.

Babe pointers

✦ **Influence is not the same as control** The idea is to have people on your side giving as much as you give, not people to act like your willing slaves. If you lose as many friends as you gain, you've got the equation wrong.

✦ **Be loyal** Loyalty pays, especially about the personal stuff. Want to keep people as friends for life? Then respect their privacy, keep their secrets and resist the urge to tell everyone about the time she wet her knickers.

✦ **Be attentive** You want influence and attention, well guess what? So do your friends. Don't make the classic mistake of making it all about you.

✦ **Be influential about the right things** It's up to your friends what they eat, wear and choose to do for a living, so don't waste your time and theirs trying to change them. If you want to have an influence on others, make it about the big stuff and the life stuff and leave the rest to them.

How to make a wedding speech

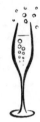 'Oh my God! Will I bore everyone to tears and make a fool of myself? Will anyone laugh at my jokes?' These are just a couple of the many, many fears that come with the knowledge that you have to make a speech in front of people who are just waiting to be entertained by your words of wisdom. Here's how to do it without having an anxiety attack.

Don't freak out

You're being asked not to talk to the nation, but to friends. All you have to remember is to keep to the point, tell people what they want to know, tell people what they need to know and express how you feel about the event. They are not expecting a stand-up comic, intellectual words of wisdom and/or a song and dance (unless these are your strong points).

Prepare something ...

... even if you don't use it. Going in cold and flying by the seat of your pants is bad news, as having 100 people suddenly look at you expectantly will give you instant stage fright. Write down some key points (you can have notes on cards if need be), role-play your speech with a friend, and be sure that you say something nice about the loving couple. Jokes about the bride's sexual past and how the groom has a big nose are best left to the best man (whom most people expect to make a pig's ear out of his speech).

Grab people's attention

In a good way – one good opener is to say, 'Pay attention, I'll be asking questions later,' or simply have something visual they can look at (blow up some baby pictures of the bride and groom, or an embarrassing but funny picture of both). Be lively – don't just stand there, move about, use gestures, smile and look people in the eye. If you're nervous, admit it, and if you're shaking, be sure to tell people it's not because you're drunk.

Breathe

Obvious, but you'd be amazed at how many people try to do difficult things without breathing. This is because when we're scared and nervous, we unconsciously hold our breath. Before you start, take three deep breaths by breathing in and letting your stomach inflate, and breathing out and letting your stomach flatten (this is the opposite of what we usually do). If your voice shakes with nerves, the trick is to breathe out and then breathe in (nerves make us do the opposite, which causes more problems) as this relaxes the throat.

Remember: it's not rocket science

It may feel like it, but you're giving a speech about two people you love. Make it heartfelt and sweet if you can't think of anything more. Drop in a few anecdotes that back your feelings up, tell them how pleased you are for them and above all, keep it short. If all else fails, just turn it into a longish toast that focuses on the fact that they are a couple in a million, and the chances are you won't be half as bad as you think you're going to be.

Babe pointers

✦ **Don't be funny** If you can't do funny, keep clear! Don't tell jokes, don't be smutty and above all don't let slip a 'funny' secret or you'll be apologising for the rest of your life.

✦ **Ad lib for immediate speeches** For spur-of-the-moment speeches just say whatever comes to mind and focus on the outcome – that is, making people feel good, rather than making a fool of yourself.

✦ **Don't be vile** It never works in a speech and neither does being horrible about someone for a laugh. If at a loss, think about how you would like a friend to talk about you at your wedding.

✦ **Relax** This is not your day, but that of the loving couple. Meaning you are not the main event, so really just focus on how it will all be over in 10 minutes, have a drink (no more than two), say your piece, and relax.

How to believe in yourself

Self-confidence, self-esteem and a strong sense of knowing what you want in life and from life are just some of the things that help you truly to believe in yourself. A daunting prospect, but something even a person lacking in all of the above can attain. Why bother, you may ask? Well, believing in yourself is about more than knowing you are good at stuff and capable of facing the tougher elements of life. It's essentially about knowing that even the bad times will pass, and everything will work out in the end. If that all sounds too rosy for you, here's how to change your attitude.

You can't control life

However, you can control your responses to it. Realising that how you face a situation is within your control is the cornerstone of self-belief. How we respond to good or bad things is a choice, meaning you can choose to face it as a learning curve or let it stamp on you. Of course, it's not always so easy to see something that is negative as a positive – but the trick here is to realise that you can and will get over it because that's what happens.

You can make anything happen

Take responsibility for all your actions, both good and bad. Life is a series of choices, which means that things don't just spiral out of our control. When things go bad it's not down to fate but the result of a series of decisions that we've made along the way. It sounds depressing but once you realise this, the upside is you can turn it around. People who have a strong sense of self-belief are those who are willing to take responsibility for what went wrong. Do this and you'll put yourself firmly back in the driving seat of your life.

Anyone can change

People change all the time simply because it's impossible to go through life and not be affected by what happens to you. If you hate your life right now this second, you can make a decision to change it (and yourself) and immediately start to be a different person. People do it all the time – think about the heartbroken who give love another chance, those who are transformed both inside and out by losing weight and even those who go through intensely traumatic events and come out even stronger than before. If they can do it, you can too.

Have realistic expectations

Having self-belief doesn't mean believing you can be happy all the time no matter what (sorry, that's called delusion). Self-belief is about knowing you are strong inside, that you can face all the aspects of life – good, bad, happy, sad and even traumatic. Yes, it helps to make good choices, and yes, it helps to do all of the above and more, but if you're determined to live a full life then you have to expect down times as well as the good times.

Babe pointers

✦ **Have attainable goals** It's our successes – whether they are passing a driving test, managing our tempers or even falling in love – that power our self-belief. If you have unattainable goals, your self-belief will flag. Have small, medium and large goals to aim for to help fuel your confidence on a daily, weekly and yearly basis.

✦ **Bin your illusions** Wishes and illusions are dangerous because they make you passive and have you living in 'What if … and when' land. If you often say, 'I'll feel better when I am thin/in love/rich,' you need to forget the future and work on what you can do now to feel good about yourself.

✦ **Life isn't always fair** It's no good asking why it isn't – it just isn't. You just have to let go of why, accept what has occurred and make a decision to get on with living.

✦ **You have only one life** So live it well – the way you want to – so that you don't waste time on things that really just won't matter in the end!

career

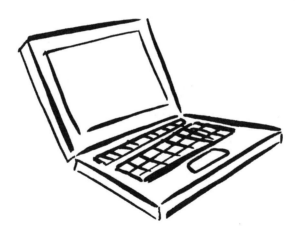

How to find a career you love

Unless you want to wake up one day and find you've been slogging away in an industry that you hate, have no interest in, or earn hardly any money from, it pays to think about what you want to do with your life. Of course, in an ideal world you'd wake up and know what you want to do, but the reality is in most people's cases it's not an inner vocation that leads them to their ideal job, but a choice. Want to feel happy about your work? Here's how.

Be realistic

A pop star at the age of 30 years? Sorry, no way. A writer/Oscar-winner after working in a video shop since you were 16? It's been done, although it's not so common. Bricklayer to doctor, shop girl to teacher, no-good-has-been to entrepreneur are all much more likely. And that's the first step to finding a career you love: reach for the stars but be realistic about your strengths, weaknesses and aims.

Think about what you love in life

This is the key to your ideal career. If it happens to be something straightforward, such as computers, your decision is made. If not, think laterally. If you like being outside, think conservation and horticulture. Love music? Then train as a radio producer or do a management course in a record shop. Love to shop? Be a buyer for a fashion chain. Love sports? Become a PE teacher or personal trainer.

Take small steps

Rome wasn't built in a day and neither will your career be. If you're eager to jump from A to X then you're going not only to lose momentum when you fail but also just to keep jumping from idea to idea. Most things in life can be achieved with a simple strategic plan that you can put into action on a daily basis. Think training, funding, apprenticeship and work experience, and then apply yourself.

Find a work mentor

Someone who is already in your dream job. If you can get to meet them, great, but if not, find out how they got there and see what you can learn from their experience.

What's your personality type?

Feeling stuck? Well, according to psychologists, there are six types of intelligence, and although we all have elements of each, we do tend to lean more towards one, which can help point you in the right work direction:

Intrapersonal intelligence You are a confident self-starter. Good for self-employment.

Linguistic You are good at verbal communication. Great for advertising, journalism and teaching.

Visual Spatial intelligence. Good for design, construction and architecture.

Interpersonal You are good at teamwork. Great for politics, teaching and management.

Physical Co-ordination and dexterity. Good for fitness work, construction and sports.

Mathematical Your power lies in logic. Good for banking, research and computing.

Babe pointers

✦ **Give yourself a time limit** Want to be a journalist but have been turned down 140 times and been waiting for a break for eight years? Time to move on and reassess your goals.

✦ **Do two things at once** Want to be a published author but need to pay the bills? You're not alone; plenty of people work a day job and follow their goals at night. Think about Stephen King who wrote his first book, *Carrie*, while working as a night janitor.

✦ **Don't listen to detractors** Be careful who you share your dreams with. Life is full of cynics who will happily tell you you'll never make it. All that matters is that you believe you can make it.

✦ **Keep trying** You may be the most talented person in the whole world, but you'll never fulfil any of your potential if you don't try – and keep on trying.

How to sail through an interview

 Are you a fly-by-the-seat-of-your-pants kind of girl? Someone who thinks on their feet, does zero preparation, and prides herself on excelling under pressure? Well, if the job of your dreams is near reach and an interview is imminent, here's the reality of what you need to know to get that job.

You do have to prepare

If you really, really want a job, you owe it to yourself to prepare. Not just for the job at hand, but for everything. Think of it like an exam, and by the time you walk into the interview, you should know details about the company, the strength of their brand (what makes them so special) and how you will fit into their set-up. Plus, if possible, their profit margins or past successes and failures!

Clothes maketh the woman

Also known as: conformity counts. There will be time later to wear pink sandals and white hotpants, but right now think neatness freak: tidy hair, subdued make-up, less jewellery, a suit or smart outfit and professional shoes and bag. Look as if you already belong to the company, and they'll rush to take you on, say the experts.

Sell yourself

As in: forget what's on your CV and what qualifications you have; instead tell them why you have; the right skills for this job and what you could bring to the company and how. One way to do this is to make an impact right at the beginning and right at the end of the interview. Being shy and bashful and then warming up is no good – you need to grab their attention right off.

Perfect your body language

Start with a firm handshake. Match the handshake of the interviewer and don't hold on too long. Next, be sure to maintain eye contact. When speaking, normal contact is between three and five seconds before you look away, but when listening, ensure you're maintaining eye contact at least 80 per cent of the time.

Deal with sticky questions

Also known as: don't be defensive. It's their job to ask you sticky questions and your job to get out of them. The key points to remember are:

When asked why you're leaving your current job, always talk about your present job and boss in a positive way. Emphasise that you're at the interview because you want to move your career upwards.

When asked about your strengths and weaknesses, don't be humble or brash about your strengths. At the same time don't list your flaws, or pretend you have none. By all means admit one, but also say how you've learnt to combat it.

When asked about the money you're looking for, either ask what they were thinking of offering, or if they already know your salary, base your answer on the market rate plus a bit extra.

Tell the truth

Finally, it pays in the long run to be honest, but there is nothing wrong with embellishing certain achievements or roles you have played in the past as long as you know you can follow through on your promises.

Babe pointers

+ **Think posture and smile** Sit up and smile as soon as you sit down; it will make you look confident, assured and friendly. Place bags to one side and hands in your lap.
+ **Be on time** Endless interviews have been flunked simply because the candidate was late. Except in the case of a natural disaster or an accident, you should always arrive with time to spare. Plan your journey and then add on an extra 45 minutes for emergencies. If more than ten minutes early, go for a coffee. Don't loiter in the reception area – it will be hell on your nerves.
+ **Have questions of your own** It's hard to appear interested if you can't think of a single question. Ask questions that demonstrate you've done your homework about the job.
+ **Elaborate on questions** Especially if the interviewer is not very good – your aim is not just to give him what he wants, but to tell him why you're so fantastic.

How to read your boss like a book

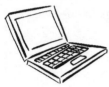

We all love to moan about the people we work for: he's stupid/lazy/a bully; she's selfish, steals my ideas and generally treats me like a slave; and so on. While some bosses are from hell, the great majority are people like you and me, with the tough task of trying to get their job done and ensure you do yours. Annoy them, sneak off behind their backs and put down their ideas and all that will happen is they'll make your life a misery. If you want to build rapport and get ahead at work, here's how to read your employer perfectly.

Learn how to read them

It doesn't take much to work out how someone thinks, acts under stress and/or copes with pressure. Knowing how to spot the different moods of your boss will get you further than you think.

Throw your antennae up and start raking in the information about them. Small observations on your behalf, such as offering to grab them some lunch when they look hassled, or agreeing with them when they're fraught, will get you far.

Work out their best time of day

Are they a lark or an owl? What time of day are they most productive and clear-minded – first thing, post lunch or late afternoon? This is the time to talk work, give them ideas and show initiative. The time they're more laid back is the time to be social and personal – mix up the two and they'll label you a slacker.

Don't be too personal

They may be quick to tell you that their wife/husband snores and hates cleaning, but don't tell *them* too much. Too much personal information can work against you at work, plus they probably just don't want to know. This is one case where they're simply allowed to spill more than you are.

Copy them

Match their voice pattern by observing the pace at which they speak (but don't copy their speaking style or they'll think you're odd). If they're a fast talker, speak slightly more slowly than they do so you look in sync. If they're a slow speaker, speak slightly faster so they speed up. It's subtle, but it's a fantastic way to build rapport. Next, work out whether they're a visual person (I 'see' what you mean), an auditory person (I 'hear' profits are low this month) or an emotional person (I 'feel' you're not happy here), and work in the same mode; for example, if they're visually led and you're putting forward an idea, paint a clear picture of it to them using visual images.

Don't be too eager to please

Initiative in your work is good, but bending over backwards to please someone isn't. Even if it works it won't make you too popular with your colleagues. Instead, do your work to the best of your abilities and then let your boss initiate the rest – after all that's their job and that's what they're getting paid for.

Babe pointers

+ **Don't fake it** It's impossible to be friends with your boss so don't try. By all means like them, admire them and get on with them, but don't try to make them socialise with you. We all have in-built fake detectors and they'll know when you're being nice to impress. Keep your compliments genuine, and offer help only when you truly think it's needed.
+ **Don't overstep boundaries** This works both ways. Just because they are your boss you don't have to answer non-work personal questions, tell them about your relationship or offer them advice on theirs.
+ **Pick up non-verbal signals** Do they always look pristine and razor sharp, or is their desk a mess of papers and cups? A person's environment can say much about their personality and what they expect from their team.
+ **Keep your distance** Never invade their personal space if you want them to respect you. If they move away as you move closer, it's a clue you're too close for comfort.

How to get a pay rise

 Want more money for shoes, to pay off your debts, or simply because you work hard and think you deserve it? Whatever your reasoning, asking your boss for more money needn't be a nervous, sweaty, nightmarish task. Here's how to ask for a pay rise without turning into a wreck.

Why do you deserve a rise?

If you don't know the answer to this before you go into your boss's office, turn back now. As any good lawyer knows, never ask a question you don't already know the answer to. Your response should be one of the following: (1) I have taken on more responsibilities than my job description states; (2) I feel I am doing the job of two people, and here's why …; or (3) According to X [find out how much others earn in your job] I should be earning more with my expertise. Here's what I can offer you, for more money.

Never, ever …

… (1) beg – maintain your dignity at all times; (2) plead poverty – companies don't want to know you have to eat to live; or (3) threaten to leave – unless you have another job in the pipeline.

Know your worth

Before you see your boss, consider your position in the company and your main bargaining tool. Are you a crucial component within a team, someone who brings in lots of business, a person whom everyone likes, or simply someone who works hard and gets results? If you're any of these, they won't want to lose you or make you feel undervalued. At the same time don't exaggerate your worth in your mind; no one is irreplaceable and you have to bear in mind the budget of the company you work for (and the rules it has about pay rises).

Be prepared to compromise

Think of what you'd be happy with and then raise it to allow for negotiation. The average pay rise is between 2 and 4 per cent, unless you're changing job roles and being promoted. It can also help to practise what you're going to say and what might happen. Ask a friend to play devil's advocate, and then negotiate your way out of it.

Choose your time wisely

It's always better to opt for a formal meeting even if your boss is your best friend and you chat regularly over the coffee machine. Better still, pick your time slot carefully: Monday morning before 11.00 and Friday afternoon (when nothing will be done until the following week) are no-gos. Early in the week is better because then you can get an answer within the week.

Know what you want before you go in

If your boss says 'No' to more money, have another plan. Either ask for more help (an assistant, a new team member) or more flexible working arrangements, or simply ask when a rise would be likely. If they say 'Never', it's probably time to look for a more rewarding job; if they says 'Soon', tie them to a three-month/ six-month deadline (in writing) and take the time to prove your worth.

Babe pointers

+ **Be reasonable** If your company has just made redundancies and put on a wage freeze you're hardly likely to get a pay rise. Either hunt for a job at a new company or hold off asking for six months.

+ **Have a five-point plan on hand** It always pays to hand over information, listing your achievements for the company in the last year, highlighting five contributions you've made and/or successes you can take credit for.

+ **Don't take it personally** If your boss says 'No', don't take it to heart - the chances are your company has strict guidelines for awarding rises. But asking never hurts and actually makes you look assertive in your boss's eyes.

+ **Don't make empty threats** Threats never work, and empty ones simply backfire. Stick to the facts and then make a decision about whether to stay or go.

How to have a productive meeting

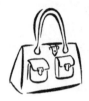 Meetings are just like parties: you don't want to go, but, boy, are you annoyed if you're not invited! And therein lies the crux of the meeting problem. Apart from the fact that most people have the attention span of a goldfish, meetings are on the whole pretty dull. If your job is to hold regular ones, here's how to make them productive and bearable for all.

What's your point?

Also known as: set an agenda. If your meetings are too casual and laid back, people will basically behave in that fashion. Make them too strict and controlling and people will do everything in their power to get out of them and/or switch off once you start talking. The key, therefore, is to know why you're having this meeting before you go into it. Ask yourself: what are you trying to get across/find out? How are you going to do this? And what's the best and most effective way to keep the meeting alive?

Get people to listen

Most people stop listening after about five minutes, so you have to keep their brains engaged. If you're not the best public speaker or a stand-up comedian, get them to think. Ask questions, set tasks, break the ice with a few non-work comments and have something for them to look at, both behind you and in front of them. It also helps to know your audience: memorise names beforehand, and use them strategically within the meeting.

Keep a firm grip on events

The best meetings are the ones where boundaries for behaviour are set, simply because within any group of people there is always the class joker ready to take control of the meeting and throw it into chaos. The best way to silence this person is to put them in charge of something, or make them give a presentation, or simply not to invite them. Don't, however, rule with an iron fist; instead, control events with your tone of voice and positive body language and, when things spiral towards mania, just be firm about keeping to the point.

Choose your time carefully

Lunchtime, and everyone will be thinking about food (and how you're taking up their free time); post lunch, and everyone will be thinking about sleep. If you want a productive meeting, the best time for people's body clocks is 11.00 a.m. This works because most people's brains will be razor sharp by then, and also lunch is on the horizon so no one will want to mess about and waste time.

Don't ramble incoherently

Want to get a message or messages across? Then be precise and don't make things too detailed and complicated. People only need to know the facts, not how you got there, what you had for breakfast and why your heel is broken. Have five key points, stick to them and reiterate them throughout the meeting.

Babe pointers

✦ **To get through a meeting** Where you sit is key in terms of an enjoyable meeting. Sit opposite a window, or anyone remotely attractive, and you'll spend the whole meeting distracted. Concentration is the key here, so sit two seats away from the speaker, preferably somewhere near an open window or near the door.

✦ **Say something** Be proactive if you're listening; it will give you valuable brownie points from management. However, make sure your comment contributes to the discussion.

✦ **Make notes** This is a great way to stay awake, and you'll be the only one to know what's going on later, because everyone else will have switched off at the ten-minute mark.

✦ **If it's going badly, say so** There's nothing more refreshing than to give people a mid-meeting break. However, don't suggest this unless you're the person actually hosting it. If you're desperate for a break – go to the bathroom!

How to manage someone

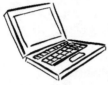 Spent years working yourself up the ladder to a position of power only to have fallen at the first post thanks to a bunch of contemptuous workers with bad attitudes and a loose idea of time-keeping? If so you need management tips, because the truth is management is one of those things everyone thinks they can do, but not everyone can. If you have trouble organising your birthdays, arranging seating plans, and getting on with more than two people at once, don't go for a management position. If that doesn't floor you, here's how to manage someone successfully.

Don't fall victim to Big Man Syndrome

Also known as: don't let power go to your head and start bossing people around. The lowly don't actually like to be reminded that: (1) you get paid acres more than them just to tell them what to do; and (2) you just want to be their 'friend'. The reality is you're the boss now – you don't get to have any friends.

Give feedback

Let people know they're doing a great job, and they will work harder for you. Keep your distance, act aloof and pull them up on the negatives without praising them for the positives and you'll soon have an unruly team who won't want to do their best for you.

A good manager is not a team player, but is also present in the workplace to give credit and recognition, and take charge of the decision-making process.

Emphasise that you're all in this together and that you're willing to do your part and they'll be more receptive to your ideas and demands.

Be firm when you have to be

Show weakness here and they'll be laughing round the coffee machine all week. Tough as it is, it's part of your job to reprimand team members. To do it correctly, your aim is to get someone to take responsibility for their actions and then problem-solve with them. Be seen to be fair by conceding things that are true, but ensure you also fight your corner in as measured a way as you can.

Take charge

People do want to be managed, because it means the buck doesn't stop with them. This means you have to take charge not only of delegation, results and personal staff issues but also of everyday things, such as meetings. Let the office joker get carried away and he'll always believe he has the upper hand. Basically, don't shy away from occasional seriousness.

Don't try to explain company decisions

There's a lot to be said for not over-explaining decisions or procedures when people you manage complain to you. In most cases trying to put forward the management side (when the facts are already out there) only escalates an argument, and makes people feel they can constantly whinge. Address the main issues, keep the decision clear and eventually people will come round. It sounds unfair, but that's management.

Babe pointers

+ **Avoid the trivial** As in: avoid getting others to do trivial personal things for you, and avoid getting involved in trivial office politics unless they're directly affecting your work.
+ **Speak to people** It sounds obvious, but you'd be amazed at how many managers don't speak to their team except to talk work issues or when problem-solving. Share a few social times – it won't kill you, and will help them to see you as 'real'.
+ **Don't fall victim to gossip** Meaning don't listen to office gossip because you never know the agenda of the person spreading the word, and at the same time don't give people anything to talk about. Keep your private life private if you want others to take you seriously.
+ **React positively to criticism** It's no fun, but you will score brownie points if you take it constructively rather than defensively. It makes people see you're human, and, who knows, you may even learn something about yourself.

How to start your own business

Have you frequently spotted a new idea or retail business and thought, 'I could do that'? If so, the idea of becoming an entrepreneur is probably at the forefront of your mind. If you're keen to go down the Bill Gates path, as opposed to that of one of the many who end up declaring bankruptcy in their first year, here's what you need to know.

Have a good idea

It sounds obvious, but many people want to go into business on their own not because they are fuelled by a great idea, but because they want to make a fast buck, think it will be fun, or can't bear the job they're currently in. So focus, focus, focus ... have an idea that is a bright spark. It doesn't have to be something unknown, and it's more likely to work if you can spot a gap in the market and give people something they simply don't yet know they want and

need (think about the coffee-shop explosion in the 1990s).

Make a business plan

A business plan is a way of logistically working out how you're going to put your ideas into action. Questions to ask yourself are: (1) how financially viable is your idea – that is, how long before your business will show a profit? (2) how will you make/create/sell and market your product? Is there a market for it? What's your budget and where is the money coming from? and finally (3) what are your cash-flow forecasts (the cash you will need to pay bills, wages and any loan)? These are the basics you need to know before you go into a bank and ask to borrow money.

Look professional

Go into any financial organisation and they will be looking at your background and planning. You should be able to show and tell are what skills you have to run your own business, your financial acumen (your grasp of money matters) and your experience in the field. Finally, they'll look for insurance – assets they can grab if you go belly up but also insurance cover for you and your business.

Have credit references

This is your credit rating based on your bank account, wages and loans you have outstanding, how long you take to pay bills, and whether you've defaulted on payments and credit cards. If you're already up to your eyes in debt, don't expect the bank readily to hand out a small fortune to you. Have this information on hand when you go in to get a loan.

Start small

In terms of both a loan and your business venture. Paying yourself a fat-cat salary and buying a flash car are not things a start-up company does. Instead, run a dummy venture for a month when you put your plans into action from your own home to see if your idea is viable. Take the project from start to finish and work out a marketing strategy alongside.

Put out feelers into the market

Otherwise known as: get out there and see if your idea is viable. Ask your prospective market what they think, or talk to people you trust working in the same field. Listen for potential areas you've missed, but above all focus on the basic idea and don't let yourself drift off on a tangent with your new-found zeal.

Babe pointers

✦ **Be prepared to work harder than you've ever done** Most new start-ups find they have to work over 100 hours per week, and that's before they start looking at accounts and planning for the future. Don't assume it will be an easy ride.

✦ **Enlist friends for help** But don't expect them to work for free. You're working for profit so they should be rewarded in some way by you, too, if you want them to remain friends.

✦ **Surround yourself with experts** You should at least have an accountant to talk to you about tax, and a lawyer for contracts. The bank will also have small-business experts on hand to advise.

How to work from home

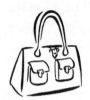

Oh, the joys of working from home! Morning TV, coffee on tap, no more early-morning alarm calls, long lunches … the list is endless. Sadly, that's not the reality. If you dream of working from home, you need a bit of planning and preparation to make sure that: (1) you get your work done; and (2) you actually enjoy it. Here's how.

Set up a separate area

You may think you can lie on the sofa with a laptop cushioned nicely on top of you, but the reality is you need a work area. By all means hot-desk, but you need designated areas that scream 'WORK' – and the sofa, bed and top of the cooker don't count. A separate area works because: (1) it immediately puts you into work mode; (2) it's somewhere to store and file all your work details; and (3) it means that working from home doesn't take over every area of your life.

Have a routine

To work from home successfully you have to have a work routine from Monday to Friday. This involves getting up at the same time every day, dressing in clothes (PJs and work don't go), turning off breakfast TV and not being distracted by domestic duties. Sadly, it's a little-known fact that people who work from home have exceedingly clean houses because they work on the I-will-do-anything-but-work principle. During your working hours, do nothing but work, and leave the rest for the weekend.

Avoid distractions

This is the major drawback to working alone and at home – there are just too many distractions and not enough reason to get motivated. The worst distractions are not things like TV and the newspaper but annoying friends calling up for a 'chat' because they're bored at work.

Endless emailing, walking to the shops for toilet rolls/milk/paper and talking to everyone from the postman to the men on scaffolding at the end of your road –

while these things may make the days go more quickly, do them too often and you'll find that, bizarrely, your work doesn't get done.

See people at least once a day

For the sake of your sanity, do, however, see at least one real person a day. If you can't make it a social encounter, join a gym or have lunch in the same café every day and practise your interaction skills before you lose all your social-etiquette know-how and your desire even to be social.

Time is different at home

You'll be amazed at how you plough through work when you're at home. Partly owing to lack of a coffee machine to wander over to, work friends to discuss soap operas with and magazines to flick through. Meaning you may feel uneasy when 2.00 p.m. comes round and all your work is done. The trick now is to go out and enjoy the whole working-from-home experience without feeling guilty.

Babe pointers

✦ **Clear all work away each night** Otherwise work will remain on your mind 24 hours a day. Your best bet is to have a work cupboard, and file and/or tidy everything every night.

✦ **Don't be afraid to say you feel lonely** It is lonely working alone – say it aloud and you'll feel better. And don't forget the pluses: no office politics, no rush hour, no being told what to do, and your own space and time to pace your work out.

✦ **Take a break at least once an hour** and every day for lunch – or else you will start reciting daytime TV and think wearing shoes is dressing up.

✦ **Start your own freelance group** For brainstorming, moaning, social interaction of the work kind and just because you can sit around and drink coffee with friends at 3.00 p.m.

✦ **Don't eat all day** Easy to do when bored/lonely/waiting on phone calls. Eat the way you would if you were at work, that is, no constant snacking. If you can't resist eating, keep the fridge clear of goodies.

How to boost your memory

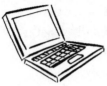

Having a good memory is as valuable as gold dust when it comes to work. Not only will it help you to remember key things such as your boss's name, where you work and what your job is supposed to be all about, but it will also boost your creative powers. People who remember things such as what they read, hear and see, are more able to make associations between them and so be more creative in the long run. If poor-memory problems are sabotaging your career prospects, here's how to help yourself.

Get to grips with your brain

The brain is like a computer: it never actually erases anything, but problems with recall occur when we stop retrieving things and so everything gets lost. It's a bit like having a pile of work papers: file them regularly and you'll know exactly where everything is. Throw everything into a large box, and even though you kind of know that the information is there, you'll have no idea how to get to it.

Exercise your head

The brain, like the rest of our body, needs exercise; that's mental and physical exercise (as well as nutrients to increase its power and boost its ability to grow). Research shows that mental stimulation keeps the brain healthy and increases memory strength. People with powerful memories tend to have a number of interests and willingly tackle challenging mental tasks.

One way to give your brain a nudge is to make yourself do puzzles and crosswords, and widen your interests, so that they cross a spectrum of things from sport to social and cultural events.

Take a supplement

The herb Ginkgo Biloba, Omega 3 and 6 essential fatty acids (found in sunflower oil, oily fish, nuts and seeds), vitamin B, zinc and iron have all been shown to have a direct effect on the brain and improve the power of memory. Reduced iron intake (common in most women) in particular has been shown to have a detrimental effect on IQ levels and cognitive function.

Visualise words

It sounds obvious, but making yourself focus on remembering is key. One exercise is to write down a list of objects, look at it for 30 seconds and then come back to it in ten minutes and see if you can remember them all. One powerful way to do this is to visualise the objects as you try to remember them. Try imagining trigger pictures against things to serve as memory nudges when remembering; for example, your best friend's new boyfriend is called Jack – recall the nursery rhyme as you say his name for the first time, and you'll always be able to remember his name.

Babe pointers

+ **Exercise your body** Thirty minutes of exercise a day can boost brainpower simply because exercise improves the heart's ability to pump blood around the body. The areas of the brain that control intellectual ability and memory benefit from improved blood flow. Exercise also boosts your metabolic rate, which helps reduce stress and improves recall.

+ **Boost your intellectual quota** If you never read, don't really have to problem-solve in your job, and never have a discussion or debate about anything more serious than what you had for dinner, you need to exercise your brain more frequently. Read more books and newspapers, listen to debates on TV, have an opinion and learn to express it.

+ **Don't be lazy** Again, recall gets easier the more you try to remember things; giving up as your brain tries to focus on something just makes your mind lazier. Create strong pathways to memories, by concentrating and focusing on what you're trying to remember.

+ **Eat a healthy diet** For good mental flexibility you need to have a healthy intake of food. For alertness you need to eat plenty of green vegetables, fruit, lean meats and nuts.

How to get ahead

 We may no longer be in the power-crazed world of the late-20th century, but it's still OK to want more from your job. However, getting ahead isn't as simple as it used to be. Apart from climbing all over your workmates to get to the top, here's how to get noticed by your bosses.

Let everyone know you're ambitious

Say it loud and say it clear, otherwise some other little upstart is going to get in there before you and ruin your chances of getting ahead. Contrary to popular belief, there's nothing wrong with saying you're ambitious and want more. In fact, hide your desires, and you'll be not only the last to hear when a promotion does come up but also the last in line.

Be proactive about everything

This doesn't mean be a brown-noser, but take the initiative when working. Being too laid back could deprive you of valuable chances to promote yourself and progress your career. So volunteer for new projects, offer insights into old ones, come forward with new creative ideas and generally get as involved as you can with the workings of your company. At the same time, think social commitments for the company: organise something – a party, a lunch, even a company newsletter.

Don't be a complainer

It's good to be vocal about your concerns but don't be the person who complains every time a new idea is put forward. You may think you're being realistic but your boss will label you as the office troublemaker. Phrase your criticisms in a constructive way, so you'll be viewed as a fixer rather than a meddler.

Raise your profile

You may be a fantastically hard worker who is at the centre of every project. However, if you don't remind key individuals of what you have done, your role will be quickly forgotten. At the same time, stay visible – make sure you're at key work social events and that you're proactive in meetings. Increasing your influence within the office should be your aim, but don't imagine you have to swing from the rafters to achieve this. It's the very basic work attributes that register as commitment in a manager's eyes. Be on time, be prepared, meet your deadlines and be dependable, enthusiastic and, of course, approachable.

Think laterally

If you work for a top-notch company the chances are you're up against people who are as smart and as canny as you are. The trick to getting ahead of them is to think laterally. Search for ways in which you can make an impact that's slightly off centre. Use knowledge you have from different areas to suggest a new way of approaching clients (such as talk to their PAs), or for selling ideas (perhaps focus on how the big brands sell their ideas), or even for bringing the company closer together. You'll also be amazed at what reading a variety of newspapers will do for your intellect and what you can then bring to the work table.

Babe pointers

✦ **Be specific about goals** About where you want to be in six months, a year, and two years from now, and set up a plan of action on how to get there. Remember: if you don't have your future mapped out, how are you going to know where you're going?

✦ **Don't be fooled by setbacks** Setbacks are just steep learning curves. Use them to learn from your mistakes by asking your boss where you might have gone wrong.

✦ **Don't be ruthless** Nastiness has a way of rebounding on you especially in work situations, so avoid stepping on others, stealing ideas and generally acting like a double agent for a few more brownie points.

✦ **If all else fails, see a careers adviser** Sometimes you can do all of the above and more, and still a company won't notice your amazing qualities. If that happens, don't stick around – answer the job adverts and find some bosses who do recognise greatness when they see it!

miscellaneous

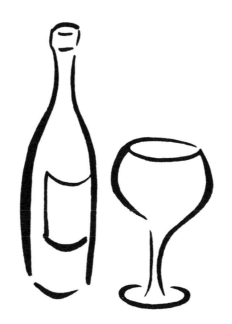

How to beat the mid-afternoon slump

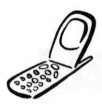

We all know the feeling – it starts with a yawn, then a stretch, then a few more stifled yawns, and then your head starts to feel heavy and your limbs flop helplessly by your side. Words swim before your eyes and that essential report seems less, well, essential. Afternoon fatigue happens for a variety of reasons, but the main cause is fluctuating blood-sugar levels in the body, which cause energy highs followed by those interminable lows. To stop snoozing and help keep your job, here's what to do.

Avoid big gaps between your meals

If you skip breakfast, starve yourself and then wait too long for lunch, too much insulin will be released to combat low sugar levels in the body when you do eventually eat. Eat little and often during the day, and never wait more than three hours before you eat something.

Eat a healthy breakfast and lunch

If you've skipped breakfast or eaten carbohydrates all morning, the result will be fatigue. The secret is to eat breakfast. Try to eat complex carbohydrates, such as oats or rye breads, and a wide variety of vegetables and fruit. An ideal breakfast would be porridge oats, or fruit and yoghurt, and/or peanut butter on rye bread. A good lunch is chicken, a Caesar salad and/or a tuna salad. For those reaching for an afternoon snack – beware of chocolate and crisps – opt for nuts, yoghurt or even a piece of fruit.

Fill up with water

If you're exhausted, it's also wise to think about what you're drinking. Research shows that one in five of us consumes too little water throughout the day – bad news for our bodies when the current recommendation is 1.5 litres (2½ pints – eight to ten glasses).

Drink less coffee

The caffeine in coffee and fizzy drinks is a stimulant that initiates an 'express delivery' of energy to the body, causing a parallel express low with a nice dose of irritability thrown in. If you really can't give it up, cut down and drink it before lunch to stop your body crashing.

Have a ten-minute power nap

Not practical at work, but achievable if you work from home, and a sensible idea as a mid-afternoon slump is a natural part of the body's normal energy rhythms. However, take only ten minutes – any more and you'll end up in a deep sleep and any chance of waking up refreshed, or with your job profile still high, will be low.

Get moving

Instead of sleeping, push yourself to be active, because physical activity will rev you up, stretch out cramped muscles and rejuvenate you. Sitting slumped over your desk all day equals bad posture, which in turn equals shallow breathing and accompanying tiredness.

Babe pointers

✦ **Talk to someone** Staring at a computer screen will only induce sleep if you're tired. Get up and speak to someone, call up someone for a quick chat, do something physical, such as filling up the photocopier. The aim is to activate your brain, not lull it into sleep.

✦ **Don't eat lunch at your desk** Not only is it not a proper break but also it induces a mid-afternoon slump through lack of exercise. A brisk ten-minute post-lunch stroll is best, not only for digestion but also for energy.

✦ **Schedule meetings in the morning** Also known as: know your energy lows. Tasks that need high concentration levels should be scheduled for the morning, not the afternoon, when your mind can't attach to the subject at hand.

✦ **Avoid quick fixes** Pick-me-ups work for only 15 minutes – so a coffee and a chocolate bar, although good fast fixes, aren't good choices if it's only 2.30 p.m. and you have three hours left at work.

How to get out of debt

 Love to shop, shop and shop? Do you have more shoes than books and more books than floor space? If so, you're probably in debt. Studies would have us believe that the average person owes around a third of what they earn each year spread over credit cards, overdrafts and store cards. If you feel nervous when you put your card in an ATM machine, and avoid opening bank statements, and if you live on the breadline a week before your wages are due, then you need to get out of debt, and fast. Here's how.

Think where your money goes

Acknowledge that you have a problem and your problem is about continuously living beyond your means, that is, you're spending too much. Like endless snacking when you're trying to lose weight, not knowing how much you are spending on a day-by-day basis will keep you knee-deep in debt for life. To focus your efforts on getting into the black, start keeping daily accounts of what goes in and what goes out.

Don't panic

Your debt will not go away if you ignore demands for money and stick your head in the sand. Credit companies get aggressive when they think you're ignoring them, so don't avoid their letters – call them up instead. If you tell them you're having problems and need their help, they'll stop sending you threatening letters and will actually help you set up a repayment plan. At the same time speak to the bank about what your best plan of action is.

Have a repayment plan

To get out of debt you don't have to win the lottery, but you can create a repayment plan that's based on real figures. There's no point in trying to pay back a large portion each month if you're left with only a meagre amount a week to survive on. You will be doomed from the start and your plan will last about two weeks. Start by allotting money for your essentials – utilities and repayments that you make each month, even if it's the minimum amount required. Next, factor in socialising (within reason) and shopping (only food, necessities and work clothes) and then look at what you have left. This is the money to use to pay off debts.

Have a long-term plan

One good option is to consolidate all your debts into a loan and then concentrate on paying just this off. If you are serious about this, it also means cutting up your credit and store cards once you have cleared the debt with your loan (as for most people a zero balance is too tempting to contemplate). This is a long-term strategy that can seem daunting at first, but it's a great way to get out of debt.

Live within your means

Also known as: find a lifestyle, don't try to buy one. Living within your means not only is the secret to happiness but also will keep your spirits up and stop you waking at 3.00 a.m. worrying about the state of your cash flow.

Babe pointers

◆ **Withdraw money on a weekly basis** Make only one cash run a week and then look at how much you're spending out on everyday things like coffee, newspapers and treats.

◆ **Get rid of store cards** They have staggering interest rates and a very firm pay-back policy.

◆ **Have a budget for everything** And stick to it. Forget the treat mentality – you're not paying off a fine, you're paying off a lifestyle you've already enjoyed. This means you should have a budget for essentials, socialising and shopping; sorry but it's called pay-back time for a reason.

◆ **See the experience as a challenge** It's depressing being in debt, so if you're going to be on a financial diet, see the positive in it. Better still, you're looking at a future where you'll actually start having money, rather than owing it.

How to get a bra that fits

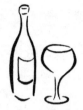 There's a reason bras come in all shapes, sizes and cup styles. Apart from the obvious point that none of us is made the same, it's impossible to tell by looking exactly what you measure or what shape bra would best suit you. Little wonder then that statistics show that 75 per cent of women wear the wrong bra size! To get the right look, think of a bra as the support structure for clothes – if you have one that bows and sags or one that binds you too tightly, you're asking for your clothes to look crumpled and baggy. Here's how to get the perfect fit.

Get measured

Use a tape measure to take a well-fitting measurement under your boobs (as in snug-fitting but not so tight-fitting you can't breathe while you're reading the size). Now add 13cm (5in): this is your band size – the part that goes round your back.

Now take a looser measurement around the fullest part of the breast. For every 2.5cm (1in) this measurement is over your band size, go up one cup size (2.5cm/1in over and you're an A cup, 7.5cm/3in over and you're a C cup, and so on).

Try on lots of bras

This is essential because no two bras are alike even if they both say 34B, plus there are half-cups (for women who are fuller at the sides of their breasts), full cups (for when you're full at the front) and balcony cups (when it's all a bit more equal). There are bras that push you in and up (think killer cleavage), minimisers that spread you outwards to make you look smaller, and Wonderbras that give the appearance of wondrous breasts when you actually have none.

Test the bras

A well-fitted bra should sit flat against your ribcage (that is, the central part of the bra should lie flat and not gape). The straps should lie taut against your shoulders and back but not fall down or dig in, and there should be no bulges around the edges, back or front of the bra cup. Remember: a bra that fits shouldn't cut off your air supply, dig into your shoulders or poke you in the sides of your breasts. The band under your breasts should be tight enough that if you slide off the straps, the bra will still support you. If the central part of the bra and the cups don't lie against your chest, go down a cup size. If your breasts are spilling forth, go up a cup size (sometimes from a D to a DD is better than from a D to an E). If the cup bags at the front, or wrinkles when you look down, go down a cup size.

Babe pointers

✦ **Buy a sports bra** Research shows that half of all women don't wear a proper sports bra when exercising; this is bad news if this is you because a lack of support will do you more damage than nipple burn. According to the experts, even if you're small-breasted and doing only gentle exercise, you can still do long-term damage to your breast ligaments. The good news is tests show wearing a sports bra reduces breast movement by as much as 56 per cent, which will help keep you both perky and fit.

✦ **Have more than two bras** Bras lose their elasticity when they are washed, so make sure you have a number of bras and keep swapping which ones you wear so that your underwear stays firm for longer.

✦ **Stock up on your favourites** Bra manufacturers, like shoe manufacturers, bring out new designs all the time, so if you find a bra you love, buy two or three, in case they stop making them.

✦ **Get measured regularly** Especially if you gain or lose weight, get pregnant, have a baby, or lose inches through exercise. Like clothes sizes, bra size needs to be reassessed every six months.

How to be ballsier

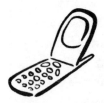

Ballsy women – don't you just love them? Hard-talking, wisecracking femmes fatales whom you'll never find crouched in a corner hiding from the crowd or sobbing into a hanky over a useless man. These women are gutsy with a capital 'G' – and the good news is you can be one of them, too. Of course, you may currently cringe at the thought of public speaking, and curl up in embarrassment about having to ask out a fantastically good-looking guy, but the truth is that somewhere inside you there is a ballsy female fighting to get out. Embrace her, because it just doesn't pay to be wimpish in this day and age. So if you're sick of being intimidated, ignored and generally walked over by friends, colleagues and people you don't even know, it's time to stick up for yourself, and here's how to do it.

Remember, no one's born with confidence

Even the gutsiest woman had to earn her stripes by practising her ballsy persona and teaching herself to speak up and speak out. The good news is that the best way to be bold is to act bold – that is, fake it to make it. Act fearless, and people will assume you are – and eventually you'll feel it too. To help yourself, start small in the ballsy stakes; after all, it takes a hardy woman to go from a fear of public speaking to speaking in front of 300 people in one jump. The key here is to take baby steps. If you hate the thought of speaking aloud, push your limits every day: speak up at meetings, interrupt when you disagree in a conversation, get used to being out there and outspoken in daily situations, and eventually your fear will decrease.

When scared, take a breath

Being ballsy is hard work, and part of it is down to the fact that it's downright scary stuff. When you're afraid, and the adrenalin courses through your veins, the trick is to quash your impulse to retreat or to talk really fast. Broadcast your courage by learning to match the voice speed of the person you're talking to, leaning in towards them and maintaining a steady voice by breathing properly (the voice cracks when you breathe too shallowly).

Control your voice

Being ballsy is not just about what you say; it's in your tone of voice and the words you use, too. Try not to do that annoying lift at the end of your sentences (it sounds as if you need reassurance from the person you're speaking to, and is distinctly unballsy). Instead, bring your voice down at the end, as it sounds more authoritative, and be straight about what you're saying. Finally, raise your energy levels as you do all this. Standing up helps, as does smiling, because it boosts your enthusiasm and generally makes you feel geared up for what you're doing.

Babe pointers

+ **Ballsy is not the same as rude** Stand up for yourself, but don't do it by standing on people or making them look small. Ballsy means you're upfront, not up your own bottom and aggressive.

+ **Have fun with it** You can be ballsy anywhere, not just at work and in confrontational situations. Try it when you're out flirting, use it to make new friends and make it part of your charm routine.

+ **Watch your body language** You might sound ballsy, but you'll look more defensive than courageous if your body language says the opposite. Remember, 55 per cent of our signals to other people come from body language, so make sure yours matches your attitude.

+ **Think bravado** Too scared to get ballsy? Well remember it's all about appearance – throw in some brave gestures and positive stances and people will simply assume you're ballsy and read you that way.

How to complain

We're a nation of complainers. We like to rant and rave and get mad, but generally it's all behind closed doors, because in reality most people feel it's just not polite to lose their temper, even if someone deserves it. Complaining is about a sense of righteousness, the feeling that overcomes us when we think we've been treated unjustly or rudely and as if we were nothing. It also happens when we feel we're being fobbed off and ignored. If you've ever been the recipient of appalling service, here's how to get your complaints in.

Assert yourself

Being assertive doesn't mean going ballistic with rage, turning bright red and SHOUTING at the top of your voice. The key here is assertiveness and not aggression. Get the two mixed up and you'll either find yourself being manhandled by security and/or end up with bigger problems than a complaint. The answer, therefore, lies in being constructive. First, make sure you're speaking to someone who can help, and secondly, make sure you have all your evidence in place so you can get your message across quickly.

Don't be self-conscious

Remind yourself you have a right to complain if you've been treated badly and/or have bought something that has fallen apart. Others may think you're making a fuss about nothing, but if you feel hard done by you have a right to say your piece and stand up for yourself. Always speak calmly. If you speak too quickly and let yourself get upset, your words will come rushing out and your complaint will get lost in the confusion.

Work out what you want

This is essential because no one can take away your anger if you don't know what will make you feel better. Are you looking for an apology, compensation, a refund and/or further action? Plus, is what you want equal to the complaint? It's no good wanting your meal for free if all that happened is the bread basket didn't arrive on time. On the other hand, having someone be rude to you does require an apology, not an off-handed attempt to make you feel better.

Know your rights

Of course, in knowing what you want it helps also to know your rights before you start shouting refund, money back and credit note. If your complaint is about something you've bought (including food) and is genuine, you do not have to take a credit note or choose something new. On the other hand, if you just don't like the shoes any more, you are not entitled to a refund (although some shops will give you one), but are often given the chance to swap goods.

Don't be afraid to go higher

If you're not getting the service you want and/or you're not getting anywhere with the person you're speaking to, don't be afraid to go higher up the chain of command. Ask for the head-office number and/or customer services, take the name of the person you have been speaking to, and make sure you have proof of purchase with you. As energising as it may be to rant endlessly at the same person, it actually gets you nowhere, plus it leaves you feeling even more aggrieved and no nearer your goal.

Babe pointers

+ **Check before you shout** Also known as: know the facts before you complain.
+ **Don't get mad, get even** Recounting a humiliating story over and over just takes away your sense of power.
+ **Don't turn into a complainer** Complaining is addictive, and once you get good at it, it can be tempting to have a go every time something goes wrong. Choose your battles wisely.
+ **Move on** Sadly, we live in a world where people are rude, stupid and sometimes downright horrible. It's a waste of your day to be fighting about their issues; fight only for yours.

How to get a flight upgrade

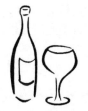 Sick of being squashed in economy, legs rolled up around your neck, someone's elbow in your side and a foot in your back? Dying to see what's behind the curtain that divides the riff-raff from the rich, but without having to pay out your life savings? Well there is a way and it's called an upgrade – the amazing feat of getting to fly like a celebrity without actually being one. Here's how to wriggle your way into a top-class seat.

Travel on your own

Sorry, but you're more likely to get a first-class or business seat upgrade if you are on your own, because it's single seats that are usually left empty. Travelling with kids certainly won't get you very far, as someone who's spent a few thousand on their ticket or is planning on doing some work on board doesn't want a child seated next to them for a flight.

Look smart

People pay a lot for first-class fares so they don't want to be seated next to someone who looks like they just fell through a hedge backwards. Also, think minimum hand luggage (no one's going to upgrade you if you're carrying carrier bags with home-made sandwiches or a massive rucksack). Make sure your check-in luggage is also smart – if it's tied with duct tape you're more likely to get an NSU on your ticket (not suitable for upgrade) than an SFU (suitable for upgrade).

Be polite

OK, so it's your honeymoon/birthday/ inaugural flight – but being a smartass, pushy, rude and/or loud and demanding will only get you a seat near the toilets at the back of the plane. While the above reasons do sometimes get you nearer the front of the plane, upgrades are at the discretion of check-in staff – annoy them and they won't do you any favours.

Become a frequent flyer

Airlines reward loyalty, especially now when everyone is more picky about with whom they fly. Show them you're a gold customer by always choosing them and you can buy an economy fare and use your free miles to upgrade to a first-class ticket at check-in.

Fly off-peak or at the busiest times

Off-peak means at those weird times when no one else wants to fly, such as during term time, when it's hurricane season at the place of destination and on days of the week and at times of day when no sane person would fly. Saturdays, Christmas Day, midday and late evenings are times when you won't see many business travellers (but lots of competitors for economy seats). This means you're more likely to be bumped upwards.

Don't fly on a cut-price airline

They don't have first class or business – meaning you'll have to sit with the riff-raff.

Babe pointers

- ✦ **Volunteer to be bumped** This is your best chance of being upgraded. Choose a flight that you know is going to be busy – usually the last flight out at a reasonable hour – and when you're at the gate, tell the check-in people you're willing to be bumped if the flight's full. This way you'll get not only compensation but also an upgrade to first class on the next flight out (as long as you weren't on a stand-by ticket).
- ✦ **Just ask** Be discreet and polite, as no one will upgrade you if you're surrounded by 100 passengers.
- ✦ **Make the best of economy** Secure the best economy seat instead of pushing for an upgrade.
- ✦ **Confirm your seats prior to flying** Use this as a chance to ask about your chances of an upgrade.
- ✦ **Don't be offended if they say 'No'** There is a strict pecking order for upgrades: they are often given to celebrities, people paying full fare and honeymooners, over regular passengers.

How to stay fertile for longer

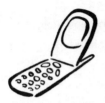 Baby Gap may not yet be your shop of choice, but it's likely that somewhere down the line it will be. However, with experts now saying one in ten couples have fertility problems due to lifestyle factors, it pays to maximise your chances of conception before you even start your plans to conceive. This means looking at a your lifestyle choices. To help you reap baby-friendly benefits, here's what the experts suggest.

Change your diet

The food you eat has a direct impact on every cell of your body, which is why a healthy diet is so important in order to conceive and give birth to a healthy baby. For this reason, it pays to 'spring clean your system' and correct nutritional deficiencies.

Diet musts

Eat a wide range of fruit and vegetables This will add essential fibre to your diet, which reduces excess oestrogen levels, and will help clear out old hormone residues.

Eat more nuts, seeds and oily fish Essential for Omega 3 and 6 essential fats, which are vital for hormonal balance, and selenium – a powerful antioxidant for optimum fertility.

Add soya to your diet in the form of tofu or soya milk Soya is classed as a phyto-oestrogen, which means it contains substances that act like hormones. This has been shown to balance the sex hormones and prevent heavy or long periods, which can affect fertility.

Quit smoking and cut your alcohol intake

Cigarette smoke in particular has been shown to decrease a woman's fertility levels by as much as 50 per cent. This is because people who smoke have high levels of cadmium, a heavy toxic metal that stops zinc (essential for fertility) from being absorbed into the body. Cigarette smoke also increases the risk of miscarriage, stillbirth, and placental damage. Alcohol, meanwhile, has been shown to poison sperm and damage ova before conception has even taken place. The most extreme effect of alcohol is demonstrated by the fact that 80 per cent of chronically alcoholic men are sterile, and alcohol is a common cause of impotence.

Maintain a healthy weight

Weight is important on both sides of the coin. A low body weight, with low body fat, lowers fertility because ovulation is hindered. Research also shows dieting and over-exercising interfere with the balance of hormones in the body, making it harder to conceive. Being overweight also lowers fertility, and losing just a small amount of weight can reverse this and stimulate ovulation as well as increase your chances of pregnancy.

Babe pointers

+ **Have a healthy sex life** Research shows that the more enjoyable the sex, the more likely you are to retain active sperm. This is because the contractions caused by an orgasm draw in more sperm, and arousal makes the vagina less acidic, allowing the sperm to survive for longer.

+ **Take a sexual health test** In 85 per cent of cases of sexually transmitted infections there are no symptoms, which means many women have an STI and don't even know about it. Get tested, get cleared and then use a condom!

+ **Get your man in on the act** Infertile men are often deficient in the antioxidant selenium, which helps make healthy sperm. Get him to take a supplement that gives him 100mcg a day. Also keep him active, reduce his alcohol intake and boost his levels of zinc, which is also essential for healthy sperm.

+ **Relax** Stress hinders your well-being, so if you're tired all the time, anxious, irritable and generally unable to sleep or function without help, then you need to learn to relax, so your body has a chance to get pregnant. Try yoga, meditation, Pilates, or even just spend more time lying on your sofa watching TV.

How to sleep like a baby

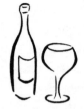

Anyone who questions the idea of beauty sleep should try talking to new mothers, anyone with insomnia or people deprived of seven hours of sleep a night. If you wake up feeling tired (and it's not due to what you've eaten), regularly get told you're irritable and moody (and it's not your personality) and have the look of someone who parties all night (and obviously haven't been), it's likely you need more sleep. Endless studies show that if you want to look good, have bags of energy and feel happy, all you need is more sleep in your life. On average 80 per cent of people have a sleep deficit, meaning they need more sleep each night. Seven hours is the norm; any less and you're going to feel horrible. Here's how to get more zzzs in.

Get rid of your problems

Surprisingly, while a good night's sleep is essential for good mental health, good mental health is also essential for a good night's sleep. It's a horrible catch-22 situation, so if you're loaded up on problems, anxious and fretting, the chances are you're not going to be able to sleep because these emotions will over-stimulate your brain. If you're lying there tossing and turning with anxiety, get up, scribble all your woes down on paper, and then literally throw your worries away. This works on the 'better out than in' principle as it clears your mind for sleep.

Wind down before sleep

Difficulty in falling asleep can also be due to anxiety, or stress of a positive kind: excitement. However, stimulants, such as caffeine (found in some medications, coffee, tea and diet drinks, to name but a few), and lifestyle factors, such as partying too hard, can also heavily influence a sleep problem. Help yourself by not drinking heavily. Also don't watch TV in bed. Research shows that the light from the TV can wreak havoc on your sleep cycle by over-stimulating your mind and increasing the likelihood of insomnia. Your best bet is to have a 45-minute winding-down period.

Keep regular hours

Remember, it's critical that you go to bed and wake up at the same time every day, as this forces the body's internal clock to stay in sync. Living it up all week and oversleeping at weekends in particular leads to Sunday-night insomnia and Monday-morning fatigue.

Think about your sleeping habits

Your sleep problems could well be down to your bed, your partner or your breathing pattern. The bed, because too hard or too soft a mattress will wake you up every time you stir in your sleep. Partners, because they snore and/or have a different body temperature in bed to you. The solution: a bigger bed or a snoring remedy. And finally, you could be suffering from a condition known as sleep apnoea – where you stop breathing as you sleep and so wake three or four times a night without knowing. If you're waking up with a sore throat, this could be the problem – see your doctor for help.

Babe pointers

+ **Do some exercise** Research from the University of Arizona shows that early-evening exercise will cause your body temperature to drop a few hours later and help make you drowsy before bed.

+ **Try vitamin B12** Studies in Japan and Germany have found that vitamin B12 (one egg a day is all you need) can aid sleep quality, as it has a direct influence on melatonin – the hormone that helps regulate sleep.

+ **Seek counselling help** Especially if you're battling unexpressed fears or suffering from post-natal depression. See your doctor for help, advice and a referral to a counsellor.

+ **Think about your pre-bed activity** A cool environment (around 16°C/60°F) improves sleep, as does a small snack before bed that isn't too high in fat and doesn't contain caffeine. Think warm milk, a mug of hot chocolate, and so on.

How to save a life

Knowing how to administer first aid is one of those things we always promise ourselves we'll learn but never really get round to, often until it's too late. Once you have rung the emergency services (or asked a bystander to do it) and checked any danger around you, here's what you should know if someone keels over in front of you.

Do your ABC

After trying to rouse them with questions, your first step should be to check that their **Airway** is clear. Do this by tilting the head backward and lifting the chin (this is the number-one way to save someone's life, as most people die because their airway is blocked). Secondly, check for **Breathing**. Is the chest moving? Lean forwards and listen – can you hear breath sounds or feel breath on your cheek? Now check the **Circulation** – feel for a pulse at their neck.

Resuscitation

Hopefully the emergency services will have arrived but if not, you will need to try to resuscitate the person. Pinch their nostrils together and hold their jaw open by pulling open the lower jaw. Take a deep breath and place your lips tightly over their mouth (so no air can escape) and breathe out for two seconds. Then take another breath and repeat.

Chest compressions

If they are still not breathing, start chest compressions: place your hands where the ribs meet the chest bone and, with your arms straight and your hands locked together, press down. The aim is to help force blood to circulate; the movement is harder than you think because you have to move the chest about 4cm (1½ in), which takes a lot of effort. Release the pressure, and repeat about once a second. Don't worry if you crack a rib – you're trying to save their life. Repeat 15 times, and then go back to mouth-to-mouth, and repeat.

Recovery position

Once they have started breathing again, place the person in what's known as the recovery position (unless there has been a spinal injury). Assuming the casualty is on their back, bend the arm nearer to you into a 'stop' position (palm up and at a right angle to the body). Bring the arm further away from you across the person's chest and place the back of their hand near their opposite cheek. Now pull the far leg into a bent position over the body. Then pull the knee and the upper body towards you so the person rolls forwards on to his or her side. Tilt the head backward to maintain an open airway and bend the upper leg at a right angle so that it helps support the body.

Wrap them up

If a person hasn't stopped breathing but looks as if they are going to pass out, it's essential to help them immediately. Prompt treatment will prevent them from fainting. First, wrap a blanket, coat or a jumper around the person and make them lie down. If there is no injury to their back, elevate their legs to slightly higher than their head. This helps encourage the flow of blood to the brain, which helps prevent them from passing out. The whole time, make sure you talk to them in a calm and soothing voice. Your aim is to reassure them that everything will be OK.

Babe pointers

+ **A fit** Contrary to popular opinion, you should never restrain someone having a fit or try to put anything in their mouth; simply protect them from injury by moving objects away from them and placing a pillow under their head.
+ **Back injury** If you suspect that someone has a spinal or head injury, do not move him or her unless they are in danger.
+ **Concussion** Seek medical help as soon as possible, and don't let them get up and start doing things.
+ **Bleeding cuts** The key to remember here is RED: Rest the patient, Elevate the bleeding limb (to above heart level, to allow the blood to flow towards the heart) and then apply Direct pressure to the wound.

How to beat PMS

PMS – is it all in the mind? Not likely! There are millions of women who suffer from pre-menstrual syndrome each month and, apart from meaning breast tenderness, mood swings, weight gain and headaches, research shows that PMS is also a key factor in 40 per cent of all relationship breakdowns. While no one knows the exact cause of PMS, one suggested cause is an abnormal sensitivity to the hormone progesterone, which rises after ovulation and often leads to a reduced level of serotonin (the body's happy chemical) in the brain. If you're a sufferer of all of the above and more, you probably already know that help for PMS is often based around short-term solutions, so here are the best things you can do to feel better fast.

Don't give yourself a hard time

PMS doesn't make you paranoid but rather brings out the deep-rooted worries and fears that you usually push to the side or ignore during the rest of the month. Which means, don't give yourself a hard time about feeling blue and down. Instead, focus on how you can resolve these issues during the rest of the month. Dealing with them when they aren't lying heavily on your mind is often a good way to prevent them from affecting you during your PMS week.

Forget about PMS-related weight gain

Weight gain – some women can put on about seven pounds or more in the days leading up to their period, but the good news is that most of this is water retention and lost during a period. If you notice that you're ravenous at this time, that's also normal because the body needs an extra 500 calories a day prior to your period. Tempting as it is to get this all from chocolate, opt for healthier foods, simply to keep your blood-sugar level from dropping and to stop food cravings. Also try eating little and often (every three to four hours), to stop your sugar cravings.

Get more sleep

This is also essential prior to your period, and if you don't get enough, it is another reason why you might feel moody and blue. Part of the problem is that your body temperature fluctuates before your period, which is why one minute you can wake up feeling boiling hot and the next wake up freezing. It can help to keep a window open and layer your bedclothes so that you can throw blankets off as you sleep.

Take a nutritional approach

Research shows that as many as 50 per cent of PMS sufferers have low levels of calcium and magnesium, as well as of B vitamins and Omega 3 and 6 essential fatty acids. It sounds complicated, but you can get all of this from the right diet. Oily fish three times a week, and green vegetables and fresh fruit three times a day, is the key to feeling better fast.

Babe pointers

✦ **Take some exercise** This not only helps relieve the physical symptoms of PMS, but also encourages the release of feelgood endorphins in the brain, which act as a painkiller and help lift your mood.

✦ **See your doctor** While there is no 'cure' for PMS, your doctor can help you with the various symptoms, especially if you feel depressed and/or can't sleep.

✦ **Take evening primrose oil** This can help restore fatty-acid levels which are often low in women with PMS. Certain studies show it can help with breast tenderness and mood, although it won't help all women. Try it for at least three months.

✦ **Keep a PMS diary** This can help you see what symptoms you get regularly and the potential triggers (foods and actions). The trick is to chart your feelings 14 days before your period begins and then work out what you can do differently the following month, such as go to bed earlier, cut down on salt, alcohol and coffee.

ALSO BY ANITA NAIK

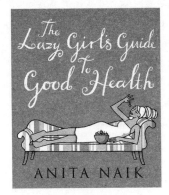

**The Lazy Girl's Guide
to Good Health**
0 7499 2253 2

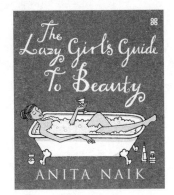

**The Lazy Girl's Guide
to Beauty**
0 7499 2399 7

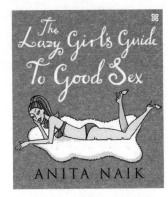

**The Lazy Girl's Guide
to Good Sex**
0 7499 2347 4

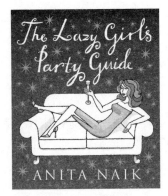

**The Lazy Girl's
Party Guide**
0 7499 2515 9

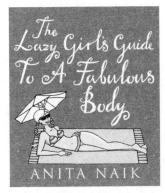

**The Lazy Girl's Guide
to a Fabulous Body**
0 7499 2432 2